D1626040

NOV 1974

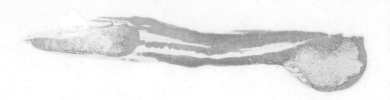

WITHDRAWN

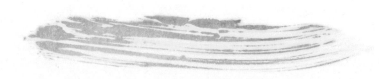

Blood Flow
and Microcirculation

PADDINGTON
COLLEGE LIBRARY,
25, PADDINGTON GREEN,
LONDON, W.2.

Blood Flow
and Microcirculation

STANLEY E. CHARM, Sc.D.

Tufts University School of Medicine
Boston, Massachusetts

GEORGE S. KURLAND, M.D.

Harvard Medical School
and
Beth Israel Hospital
Boston, Massachusetts

A WILEY-BIO-MEDICAL HEALTH PUBLICATION

JOHN WILEY & SONS, New York · London · Sydney · Toronto

PADDINGTON
LIBRARY.
512.13 18.10.77
26202
Class No. 612.13

Copyright © 1974, by John Wiley & Sons, Inc.

All rights reserved. Published simultaneously in Canada.

No part of this book may be reproduced by any means, nor transmitted, nor translated into a machine language without the written permission of the publisher.

Library of Congress Cataloging in Publication Data:

Charm, Stanley E

Blood flow and microcirculation.

"A Wiley-Bio-Medical Health publication."
Bibliography: p.
1. Blood flow—Measurement—Mathematical models.
I. Title. [DNLM: 1. Blood flow velocity.
2. Microcirculation. WG103 C482b 1974]

QP105.4.C45 1974   612'.13   73-15977
ISBN 0-471-14820-2

Printed in the United States of America

10 9 8 7 6 5 4 3 2 1

Preface

Information on various aspects of blood viscosity and its relation to flow in the microcirculation has expanded considerably over the past few years. Many investigators with a knowledge of engineering or physics have examined problems of the circulation from their respective vantage point. Their view, which differs from that of classical physiology, has brought new insight into the problems of blood flow and has demonstrated the value of an interdisciplinary approach.

It seems appropriate at this stage to gather this information and to focus attention on quantitative analyses of flow in the microcirculation. Most of the studies on which these analyses are based were carried out in *ex vivo* systems. Since there are very few data on pressure–flow-rate relationships in *in vivo* systems, it is not possible to establish how well *ex vivo* data may be applied to *in vivo* systems. In nearly all studies of flow in living systems, for example, lower resistance is noted in *in vivo* flow as compared with *ex vivo* flow (see Chapter 3). Thus there continues to be a critical need for experimental verification of the equations and models that have been developed. Such work has lagged because of the difficulty of obtaining simultaneous pressure–flow-rate measurements in small vessels.

A number of controversial issues remain to be resolved. We have selected the approach that seemed most reasonable to us. One of our major purposes is to point out methods for making quantitative estimates of flow in the microcirculation under various conditions. With all the shortcomings of these models, we believe that order-of-magnitude estimates can be made in most cases by extrapolation from *ex vivo* data. Illustrative numerical examples of calculations are presented to familiarize the reader with the mechanics of problem solving. Some of these problems may appear to be highly complex, but they are necessary to illustrate concretely the calculation method. The examples dealing with branch flow and capillary flow may fall into this category. In fact, what seems to be too complex to some readers who are trained in biology may be elementary to others who are trained in engineering. Like all marriages, the union of biology and quantitative engineering requires mutual tolerance, respect, and adjustment. The paucity of hard data and the infinite variety of biologic systems confound quantitative analysis. On the other hand, few biologists or physicians are comfortable with the requisite mathematical tools for quantitation.

A chapter on the importance of blood rheology in clinical medicine is included. The changes in viscosity and their consequences are described in qualitative terms, but it is possible to estimate the quantitative role of blood rheology in pathologic states.

We wish to express our appreciation to the National Heart Institute of the National Institutes of Health and the Massachusetts Heart Association for supporting our research, through U.S. Public Health Service grant HE-08783 and grant-in-aid 850 from the Greater Boston Chapter of the Massachusetts Heart Association.

We also thank David H. Brand for his help in writing the computer programs that appear in the appendices of various chapters. We extend our thanks to Prof. Walter L. Hughes, Chairman, Department of Physiology, Tufts University School of Medicine, for his encouragement and support. Finally, we also thank Ronald Rutchick for drawing the figures.

STANLEY E. CHARM, SC.D.
GEORGE S. KURLAND, M.D.

Boston, Massachusetts
September 1973

Contents

Blood Flow
and Microcirculation

Introduction

Chapter 1

UNDERSTANDING FLOW IN THE MICROCIRCULATORY SYSTEM requires the application of fluid dynamic principles within the framework of anatomy and physiology of the microcirculation. Simple fluid flow through a conduit is influenced by the geometry of the conduit, the roughness of the walls, and characteristics of the fluid and the forces acting on the fluid. An important characteristic of the fluid is the resistance it offers to the shearing of its molecular bonds by the applied force, whose critical properties are direction and magnitude; in some cases, time of application is also significant.

Although a general outline of the geometry of the circulation is useful for hydrodynamic purposes, special circulations exist to meet the functional needs of individual organs. The conduits for blood in man are the aorta, the larger arteries, the main artery branches and arterioles, the capillaries, the terminal veins, the main venous branches, the larger veins, and the vena cavae. The geometry and size of these vessels are noted in Table 1.1. The range is from 1.5 cm in diameter for the aorta to about 8×10^{-4} cm for a capillary. The vessel distribution and dimensions found in the bat wing are listed in Table 1.2. The greatest vessel cross-sectional area and capacity is found in the venules (Wiedeman, 1963). Although the definition of vessel size included in the microcirculation is arbitrary, here it includes terminal branches of arteries, arterioles, capillaries, venules, and terminal veins. The flow of blood in these vessels varies intermittently; in contrast with the pulsatile flow in the aorta and large arteries, however, it is not pulsed. The velocity, pressure, and blood volume associated with various vessels are given in Fig. 1.1.

Walls of all vessels except capillaries and some venules are composed of collagenous fibers, smooth muscle, elastin, and endothelial lining cells. Capillaries contain only endothelial cells, and some venules consist of endothelial cells having a small number of fibers. Larger venules contain smooth muscle (see Fig. 1.2). The walls of arteries and veins are classically described in terms of concentric zones: intima, internal elastic lamina, media, and adventitia. The adventitia and the media are the major stress-bearing components. The media contains the vascular smooth muscle. The media of an elastic artery is composed of a series of concentric elastic lamellae connected by obliquely oriented smooth muscle fibers. The muscle fibers in adjacent interlamellar spaces often run in reverse direction, giving the wall a herringbone appearance.

Unlike the aorta, the main pulmonary artery and its major branches have no elastic lamellae, the elastin having a sparse distribution. The fibers are short and separated by other slender elastin fibers terminating in clublike expansions (Harris and Heath, 1972). The major pulmonary artery has a relatively thin wall, its medial thickness being 40 to 70% that of the aorta.

Veins differ from arteries in that the former have valves; moreover, their walls are thinner, and they are often in a collapsed state. Their media consists essentially of spirally arranged smooth muscles with few elastin fibers. This

3

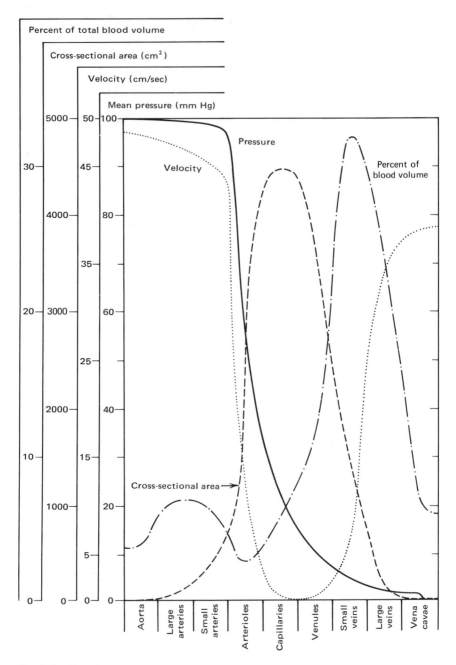

Fig. 1.1 Quantitative aspects of the circulatory system (from Berne and Levy, 1972, Cardiovascular Physiology, C. V. Mosby Co.).

Table 1.1 Geometry and Structure of Various Vessels[a]

| Vessel | Diameter (cm) | Length (cm) | Wall Thickness (cm) | Composition (%) | | | | |
				Endothelium	Elastic Tissue	Smooth Muscle	Fibrous Tissue
Aorta	2.5	50	0.2	5	40	25	30
Artery	0.4	50	0.1	5	35	40	20
Arteriole	0.005	1	0.2	5	25	45	25
Precapillary sphincter	0.0035	0.02	0.003	15	15	50	20
Capillary	0.0008	0.1	0.0001	100	0	0	0
Venules	0.0020	0.2	0.0002	25	0	0	0
Vein	0.5	25	0.05	5	40	30	25
Vena cava	3.0	50	0.15	5	25	35	35

[a] Adopted from Burton (1965).

Table 1.2 Dimensions of Blood Vessels in the Bat's Wing[a]

Vessel	Average Length (mm)	Average Diameter (μ)	Average Number of Branches	Number of Vessels	Total Cross-Sectional Area (μ^2)	Capacity ($mm^3 \times 10^{-3}$)	Percentage of Capacity
Artery	17.0	52.6	12.3	1	2,263[b]	38.4	10.1
Small artery	3.5	19.0	9.7	12.3	4,144	14.4	3.8
Arteriole	0.95	7.0	4.6	119.3	5,101	4.7	1.2
Capillary	0.23	3.7	3.1[c]	548.7	6,548	1.5	0.39
Postcapillary venule	0.21	7.3		1,727.0	78,233	16.4	4.3
Venule	1.0	21.0	5.0	345.4	127,995	127.9	33.7
Small vein	3.4	37.0	14.1	24.5	27,885	94.7	25.0
Vein	16.6	76.2	24.5	1	4,882	81.0	21.4

[a] From Wiedeman (1963).
[b] Average of individual cross-sectional areas.
[c] Calculated.

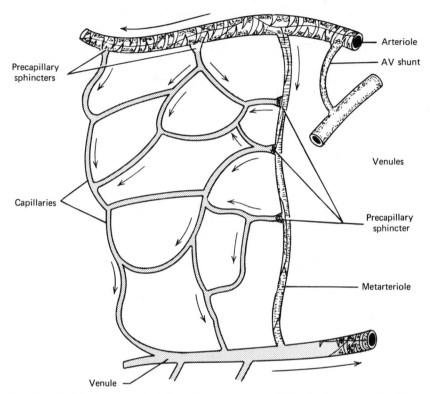

Fig. 1.2   Model of capillary bed (from Berne and Levy, 1972, Cardiovascular Physiology, C. V. Mosby Co.).

relative lack of elastin fibers constitutes the major structural difference between arteries and veins. In some medium-sized veins, the innermost muscle fibers in the media are oriented longitudinally (Ham and Leeson, 1961). Veins in the limbs have a thicker media than elsewhere, consistent with the higher hydrostatic pressures developed in this part of the venous system. In large veins there is little smooth muscle in the media. The adventitia is thicker than the media and contains both collagen and elastin fibers. Like the smaller veins, the inner layer of muscle is longitudinally disposed (Gow, 1972).

The endothelial lining provides a smooth interface between flowing blood and the vessel wall. It has been postulated that an inner lining of blood vessels, which covers the endothelial cells, consists of a fibrin film (Copley, 1953). This film is dynamically maintained, and it has been suggested that it reduces the friction associated with blood flowing in the vessel (Copley, 1960). The physical mechanism by which the frictional energy loss is decreased has not been clearly visualized; possibly, however, it influences the contact of the red cell with the vessel wall.

Vessel walls with smooth muscle are subject to nervous activity, and such vessels are capable of constricting or expanding their diameters. Capillaries on the other hand are not subject to nervous activity and respond passively to the internal pressure within the vessel. However, there may be a relatively high concentration of smooth muscle, the precapillary sphincter, at the junction of an arteriole and a capillary, and this area is subject to nervous control that regulates capillary flow. The effector mechanism for individual capillary flow regulation is now thought to be the precapillary sphincter rather than the capillary itself, as originally postulated by Krogh (Johnson, 1972).

In addition, it is possible to transfer blood from the arteriolar to venular side without passage through the capillary bed by means of direct connections known as arteriovenous anastomoses or AV shunts (see Fig. 1.2). An AV shunt contains smooth muscle and is therefore also subject to nervous control. When there is a sudden demand for blood in one part of the body, the AV shunt acts to divert blood without passage through the capillaries, from those parts not subject to the demand.

Control of flow resistance in the microcirculation ultimately resides in the vessel diameters. In vessels with smooth muscle the diameter is determined by the balance of tension in the wall and by internal pressure in the vessel. Wall tension is in part a function of nervous control and thickness of the vessel wall.

Vessels contain curves, bends, enlargements, and contractions. These variations in geometry disturb the flow pattern as it appears in a straight length. This causes an increase in flow resistance. At a bend, for example, the fluid near the inside of the bend moves slower than the fluid in the central regions, and the centrifugal force experienced by the fluid may set up eddy currents or secondary flow in the vessel. This effect on energy loss is negligible in small vessels, however.

At a vessel branch the fluid may be disturbed sufficiently to cause turbulence (i.e., random mixing). Turbulence may also be induced in straight lengths by a sufficiently high flow rate. The interaction of particles within the fluid causes additional variations in the flow patterns.

When a fluid flows past a solid, the fluid immediately in contact with solid boundaries does not slip relative to the solid boundary (e.g., a vessel wall). This

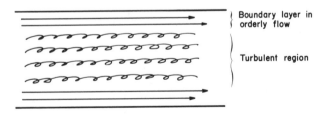

Fig. 1.3   Boundary layer in the case of turbulent flow.

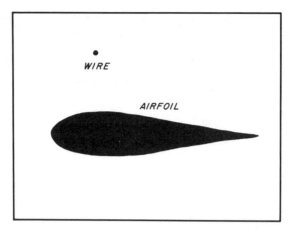

Fig. 1.4   Sphere or wire diameter producing same drag as much thicker foil.

stability is noted even with nonviscous fluids such as air and nonwetting fluids such as mercury. Between this film of absolutely motionless fluid and the moving mainstream, there is a region of flow called the "boundary layer." In the boundary layer the velocity changes from zero at the wall to a velocity unimpeded by viscous forces.

In the case of low flow and viscous fluid, the boundary layer may extend all the way to the centerline. However, in rapid flow where turbulence exists in the mainstream (see Fig. 1.3), the boundary layer offers resistance to heat and mass transfer. It is responsible for the drag on streamlined and unstreamlined shapes. For example, air exerts more drag flowing past a thin wire than it does on a much thicker streamlined airfoil (e.g., see Fig. 1.4). The reason is that blunt objects such as the wire or sphere cause rapid separation of the boundary layer, resulting in backflow and eddy currents at the rear of the objects (see Fig. 1.5). The streamlined object extends the boundary layer relatively undisturbed into the mainstream, without eddy currents and backflow, which consume energy in fluid friction and disorder (see Fig. 1.6; e.g., Shapiro, 1961). This boundary layer around cells, which has not yet been well studied, may influence cellular aggregation and may explain such important phenomena as movement of cells away from the vessel wall under certain conditions.

1.1   POISEUILLE'S STUDY

Prior to 1842 it had not been established that the movement of blood through capillaries had its origin solely in the contractions of the heart. Contemporary theories suggested that the capillaries themselves caused the flow of blood or that the cells themselves caused movement.

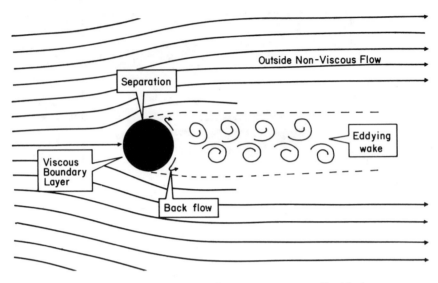

Fig. 1.5   Flow pattern at high flow rate past unstreamlined body.

Jean Poiseuille (1842), a French physician, reasoned that if lengths and diameters of the capillaries are different in various animals, and if the pressure and temperature of the blood vary in different parts of the body, light might be thrown on the problem of flow by investigating the effects on flow rate of pressure, length, diameter, and temperature. The results of Poiseuille's experiments were of a more fundamental character than he realized.

Bingham (1922) reviewed Poiseuille's work and published his results in full. Poiseuille measured the efflux times of water by the absolute method, taking elaborate precautions to ensure accuracy and using glass capillaries of various lengths and diameters which were equivalent to separate instruments. The capillaries used were elliptical in cross section rather than circular. The major and minor axes differed on the average by about 5%. Poiseuille observed that the flow rate of water is inversely proportional to length and proportional to the fourth power of the tube radius. End effects and kinetic energy corrections (discussed later) were omitted from his considerations.

Poiseuille's work merits detailed study not only for its historic interest, but also because of its bearing on questions that arise subsequently.

Hagenbach (1860) appears to have been the first to give a definition of viscosity. He established the following theoretical derivation of Poiseuille's law:

$$(1.1) \quad Q = \frac{\pi P}{8 \mu L} R_w^{\,4}$$

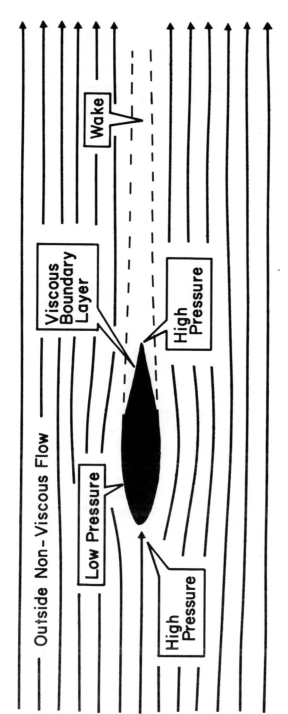

Fig. 1.6 Boundary layer around streamlined object with no eddying wake.

11

where μ = viscosity

Q = flow rate (volumetric)

P = pressure difference between entrance and exit

L = length

R_w = radius of tube

In deriving Poiseuille's law, Haganbach made four assumptions.

1. Flow is laminar; that is, each streamline or lamina of fluid moves downstream in an orderly fashion (see Fig. 1.7).
2. The layer of fluid next to the wall is stationary.
3. The velocity of each layer or streamline of fluid is proportional to force acting on it (Newtonian fluid); the proportionality constant is known as viscosity. (This is discussed in more detail later.)
4. The system is isothermal.

Poiseuille compared rates of flow of blood serum through glass tubes and through a given vascular territory, varying the viscosity of the serum by addition. It has been assumed that the laws of Poiseuille apply also to the flow of blood through the capillaries of the body. Ewald (1877) questioned this conclusion, and Hübener (1905) noted an incongruity in the flow rate of solutions of known viscosity in the organs of a frog. Lewy (1897), however, found that Poiseuille's law holds as long as no sedimentation occurs.

Poiseuille observed that a cell-free layer appeared near the tube wall under certain conditions and ascribed deviations from equation 1.1 to this effect. duPre Denning and John Watson (1900), from studies of the effect of bore size on blood flow, concluded that blood containing a large number of corpuscles did not obey Poiseuille's law if the tube diameter was less than 300 microns (μ); that is, the viscosity was apparently a function of radius for smaller capillaries. They noted an increase in viscosity with decrease in tube diameter and also observed that viscosity depended on the drawing pressure for these small tubes.

The physiologist Walter R. Hess (1910–1912) studied the flow of blood and,

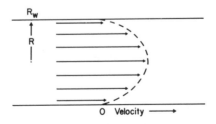

Fig. 1.7   Velocity profile for Newtonian fluid in laminar flow.

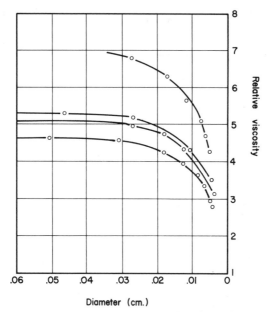

Diameter (cm.)

Fig. 1.8   Decrease in apparent viscosity of various blood samples with tube diameter (from Fahraeus and Lindquist, 1932).

noting that the measured viscosity depended on the apparatus, convinced himself that he was not dealing with turbulence. Contrary to the contention of duPre Denning and Watson, Hess concluded that it was not simply the diameter of the tube that caused the deviation from Poiseuille's equation, citing instead "cohesive forces" in the fluid.

Fahraeus and Lindquist (1929) also studied blood flow quantitatively in glass capillary tubes and found the marginal layer to be most prominent in tube diameters less than 300 μ. They noted that the "apparent" viscosity of blood as calculated from Poiseuille's equation decreased with a decrease in the tube diameter (see Fig. 1.8), in contradiction to duPre Denning and Watson. This phenomenon, known as the Fahraeus-Lindquist effect, was thought to occur in vessels. Whitaker and Winton (1935), who studied flow in the hind limb of a dog, suggested that the Fahraeus-Lindquist effect explained the lower apparent viscosity they observed in vessels as compared with glass tubes.

Another curious property of the apparent viscosity of blood appears in the observations of flow in a single tube. The apparent viscosity increases at low flow rates, but at high flow rates it approaches a lower apparent viscosity asymtotically (see Fig. 1.9).

Fahraeus and Lindquist concluded that Poiseuille's equation applies under a wide range of conditions in physiology. For example, from Fig. 1.8 it appears to

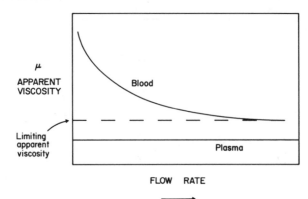

Fig. 1.9   Change in apparent viscosity of blood with flow rate. Plasma has a constant viscosity.

apply to whole blood suspensions (i.e., cell volume fraction $\phi = 0.45$) under two conditions: (a) the suspension is flowing in tubes with diameters greater than 300 μ, and (b) the flow rate is sufficiently great that the asymptotic apparent viscosity applies throughout the vessel. When there are deviations from the asymptotes in Figs. 1.8 and 1.9, deviations from Poiseuille's equation occur. Many studies have been made of the deviations of blood flow from Poiseuille's equation, including Thomas (1962), Bugliarello (1965), Haynes (1960), Haynes and Burton (1959), Bayliss (1959), Taylor (1955), Fahraeus and Lindquist (1932), Hershey and Cho (1965), and Charm and Kurland (1962).

1.2   CALCULATION OF FLOW WHEN POISEUILLE'S EQUATION APPLIES

Consider the flow in a system of vessels shown in Fig. 1.10. As in most types of flow, the flow rate Q = driving force/resistance. In this case the driving force is the pressure difference between entrance and exit of the tube or vessel, and the resistance is $8\mu L/R_w{}^4 \pi$. From an examination of equation 1.1 it is evident that a 10% change in radius causes a change of approximately 40% in flow rate, other factors being constant.

It is possible to determine the flow rate and pressure loss in each branch of the system in Fig. 1.10. Sometimes it is easier to do this by considering the electrical analog to the flow system, as in Fig. 1.11. In the electrical analog, the flow rate of electrons or the current l is related to driving force and resistance by Ohm's law, $I = E/R'_,$, where E is potential difference and $R'_,$ is electrical resistance.

Expressed in a form analogous to Ohm's law, Poiseuille's equation would be

(1.2) $$Q = \frac{P}{8\mu L/R_w^4 \pi} = \frac{E}{R'} = I$$

The total flow rate, the total pressure drop and viscosity of blood, and the diameter and length of each vessel are known. Through use of the electrical analog, it is possible to calculate the flow rate in each branch through a series of equations which involve the voltage drop E across each branch and current flow (1) around each point. From Fig. 1.11 there are 12 equations and 12 unknowns, as shown in Table 1.3. It is necessary to solve these 12 equations simultaneously to obtain the flow rate in each branch.

Table 1.3   Table of Equations for Electrical Analog of Vessel Network (see Fig. 1.11)

$$I_1 = I_5 + I_2$$

$$I_5 = I_8 + I_9$$

$$I_1 R_1 + I_5 R_5 + I_8 R_8 + I_{16} R_{16} + I_{40} R_{40} + I_{47} R_{47} = E - I_{54} R_{54}$$

$$I_1 R_1 + I_5 R_5 + I_{19} R_{19} + I_{41} R_{41} + I_{47} R_{47} = E - I_{54} R_{54}$$

$$I_9 = I_{19} + I_{20} + I_{21}$$

$$I_9 = I_{41}$$

$$I_{40} = I_8$$

$$I_8 = I_{16} + I_{17} + I_{18}$$

$$I_{16} R_{16} = I_{17} R_{17} = I_{18} R_{18}$$

$$I_{19} R_{19} = I_{21} R_{21} = I_{22} R_{22}$$

$$I_{47} + I_{53} = I_{54}$$

$$I_{40} + I_{41} = I_{47}$$

$$I_{47} = I_5$$

The solution for a simple branched flow system appears in Example 1.1 (see calculations). Note in Example 1.1 how a change in flow rate in one branch must affect the flow rate in the other branch.

The electrical analog is no better than the information on which it is founded. In the example considered, several important factors have been omitted, including the nature of the vessels themselves – they are not rigid and of uniform diameter, but are elastic and taper. Also, flowing blood does not always follow Poiseuille's equation. These points are examined later to permit the formation of a more realistic model.

1.3   FLOW RATE REDUCTION IN PRESENCE OF A STENOSIS

It has been observed that a stenosis in the aorta does not appreciably reduce circulation until 80% of the vessel has been occluded (e.g., May et al., 1963; Weale, 1967). The explanation lies in considering the circulation in terms of

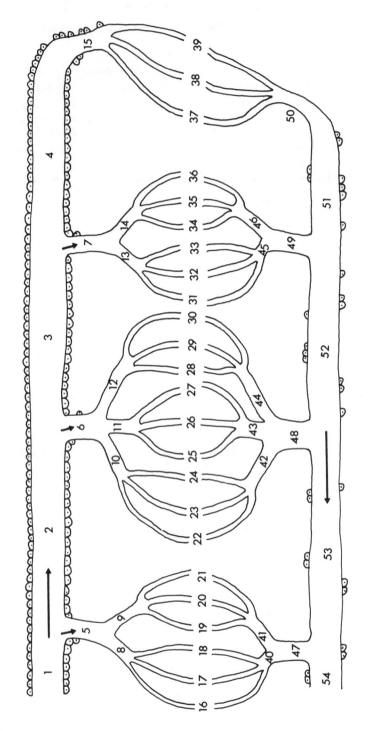

Fig. 1.10 A hypothetical vessel network showing smooth muscle controlling constriction of larger vessels.

16

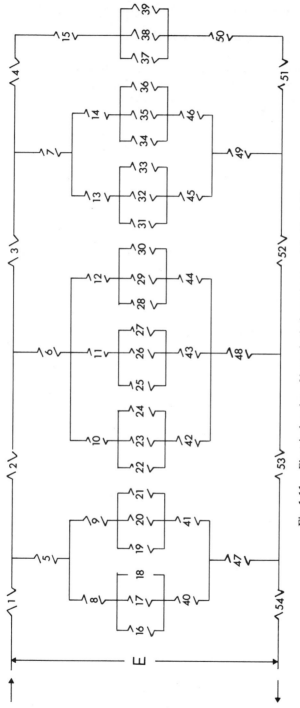

Fig. 1.11 Electrical analog of hypothetical vessel network in Fig. 1.10.

17

resistances in series; a quantitative demonstration of this phenomenon can be made with Poiseuille's equation.

To cause a reduction in circulation, the flow resistance through the stenosis must be in the same order of magnitude as the flow resistance through the rest of the circulation. The normal circulation resistance can be estimated from Poiseuille's equation. Circulation flow rate is about 100 ml/sec with a pressure difference of about 100 mm Hg and a viscosity of about 0.04 poise (P). Using Poiseuille's equations to calculate resistance, we have

$$100 = \frac{100 \times 1.33 \times 10^3}{(0.04)(8)/\pi \, (L/R^4)}$$

$$\frac{L}{R^4} = 12.37 \times 10^3$$

Flow rate in the presence of a stenosis follows the equation

$$Q = \frac{12.37 \times 10^5}{12.37 \times 10^3 + (L_1/R_1^4)}$$

Where L_1 and R_1 refer to the length and radius of the stenosis.

Consider an aorta with a radius of 1.00 cm. If a stenosis develops with a length L_1 of 1 cm, a calculated plot of flow rate and radius of the partially occluded area (Fig. 1.12) shows that the flow rate remains essentially constant until the vessel is 80% occluded and the stenosis resistance is in the same order of magnitude as the rest of the circulation. The turbulence which most likely occurs in the stenosis when the radius of free space/radius of aorta is less than 0.5 has been neglected here.

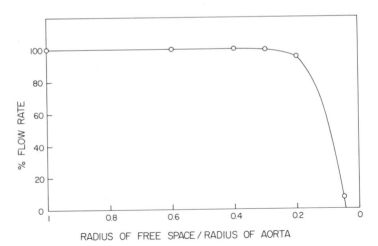

Fig. 1.12   Circulation flow rate as a function of stenosis radius.

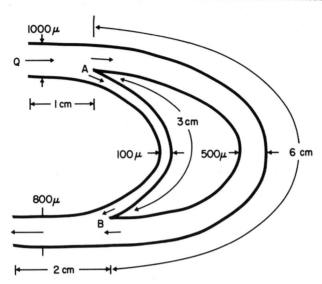

Fig. 1.13   Hypothetical vessel network with two branches; see Example 1.1.

Example 1.1

Consider the flow in the isolated vessel network appearing in Fig. 1.13. The flow rate through the system is 0.02 cm³/sec. Assuming that Poiseuille's equation applies, what is the pressure drop from point 1 to 2? The apparent viscosity of the blood is 0.025 P.

Solution

In the 1000-μ branch, pressure drop is

$$P_1 A = \frac{Q 8\mu L}{\pi R_w^4} = \frac{(0.02)(8)(0.025)(1)}{\pi(500 \times 10^4)^4} = 2.04 \times 10^2 \text{ dynes/cm}^2$$

At point A the flow divides into Q_{100} and Q_{500}. To solve for $Q_{100}, Q_{500}, P_{100},$ and P_{500}, it must be realized that pressure drop between A and B is the same irrespective of the branch through which flow takes place. Thus we have

$$P_{AB} = \frac{Q_{100}(8)(0.025)(3)}{\pi(50 \times 10^{-4})^4} = \frac{Q_{500}(8)(0.025)(6)}{\pi(250 \times 10^{-4})^4}$$

Also, $Q_{100} + Q_{500} = 0.02$ cm³/sec; thus we continue as follows:

$$P_{AB} = 0.02 - Q_{500} \frac{(8)(0.025)(3)}{\pi(50 \times 10^{-4})^4} = \frac{Q_{500}(8)(0.025)(6)}{\pi(250 \times 10^{-4})^4}$$

$$Q_{500} = 0.0168 \text{ cm}^3/\text{sec}$$

$$Q_{100} = 0.0032 \text{ cm}^3/\text{sec}$$

and

$$P_{AB} = \frac{(3.2 \times 10^{-3})(8)(0.025)(3)}{\pi(50 \times 10^{-4})^4} = 9.80 \times 10^5 \text{ dynes/cm}^2$$

or

$$P_{AB} = \frac{(1.68 \times 10^{-2})(8)(0.025)(6)}{\pi(250)(10^{-4})^4} = 9.80 \times 10^5 \text{ dynes/cm}^2$$

In the 800-μ branch we have

$$P_{B2} = \frac{(0.02)(8)(0.025)(2)}{\pi(400 \times 10^{-4})^4} = 1.3 \times 10^3 \text{ dynes/cm}^2$$

Thus

$$P_{12} = 2.04 \times 10^2 + 9.80 \times 10^5 = 1.00 \times 10^3 = 9.812 \times 10^5 \text{ dynes/cm}^2$$

In this case, pressure losses due to entering different size channels were neglected, as were kinetic energy effects, which are covered in Chapter 3. Note that constricting either branch affects the overall pressure drop in the system.

Blood Viscosity

Chapter 2

2.1 STRUCTURE OF BLOOD

BLOOD IS A SUSPENSION OF CELLS IN PLASMA. At rest, the cells form a continuous structure (see Fig. 2.1, e.g.; Charm et al., 1964). When the structure breaks under its own weight, sedimentation occurs. Evidence of such continuous structure appears when the blood structure is given sufficient support against its own weight (e.g., by the wall of a settling tube) and settling is prevented. The viscometric behavior of blood is the result of the resistance of blood structure to the forces attempting to deform it (Goldstone et al., 1970).

When a finite stress – a force/unit area – is applied to whole blood, the continuous structure breaks. The stress required to disrupt the standing structure of blood is referred to as the yield stress. After disruption the structure is characterzed by clusters of cell aggregates suspended in plasma. The aggregates in turn are made up of smaller units of cells called rouleaux or flocs. As additional stress is applied, the aggregates and the rouleaux become smaller. A dynamic equilibrium exists between the size of aggregates or rouleaux and the stress applied (see Fig. 2.2). When aggregates and rouleaux are under stress that is high enough to reduce them to individual cells, further increases in stress cannot

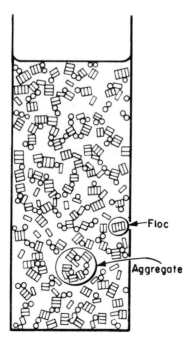

Fig. 2.1 Cell suspension at rest is a continuous structure formed from groups of cell aggregates made up of units of cells called flocs or rouleaux.

23

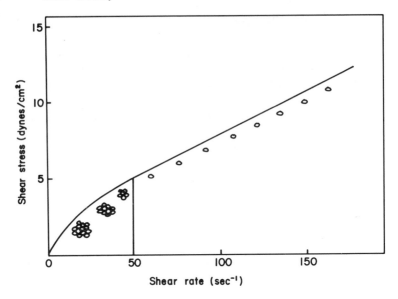

Fig. 2.2   Dynamic equilibrium between cell aggregate size and shear stress applied.

result in changes of aggregate size. As a result of dynamic equilibrium, the shear-stress—flow-rate relationship becomes a straight line at sufficiently high shear stresses (see Fig. 2.2). This "shear thinning" effect is also influenced by the deformability of the red cells.

Red cells deform under stress, becoming more elongated at high stresses. It has been suggested that this change in shape from spherical or disc to an elongated rod also relates to the shear-stress—flow-rate relationship becoming a straight line independent of aggregation characteristics (Schmid-Schönbein et al., 1972). The nature of the attraction between cells that causes these units to aggregate is still not clear. Both electrostatic attraction and plasma surface tension have been suggested as mechanisms (Fahraeus-Lindquist, 1932; Castaneda et al., 1965), as well as long rodlike molecules interlocking cells.

In a dilute suspension containing 1% cells, about 30 sec is required to achieve equilibrium when a change in stress occurs. The thixotropy or viscosity time effect here is not very pronounced at such a low concentration because the cells contribute so little to the suspension viscosity. In more highly concentrated suspensions, on the other hand, the time needed to achieve equilibrium is less. The viscosity change at low flow rates is due to changes in aggregate or rouleau size. Since large aggregates tend to structure the suspending fluid more than smaller ones, higher apparent viscosities are associated with larger aggregates.

When flow oscillates (e.g., at a frequency of 10 Hz) blood exhibits elastic properties at sufficiently high cell concentrations (greater than 20%). There is a distinction between the influence on blood viscosity arising from interactions between red blood cells and the effect that is associated with the isolated, noninteracting red cells in surrounding plasma. When cell concentrations are less than 5%, the viscous component approaches the dilute solution value (see Section 3.11: Thurston, 1972).

2.2 MEASUREMENT OF BLOOD FLOW PROPERTIES

Measurement of the relation between stress and flow is carried out in an instrument (viscometer) designed to permit analysis of the stress acting on the fluid for a given flow condition.

The principle of a viscometer can be illustrated by considering the following model: a fluid is placed between two parallel plates (see Fig. 2.3). A force F

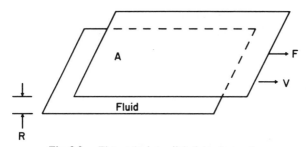

Fig. 2.3   Theoretical parallel plate viscometer.

applied to the top plate is sufficiently small that the velocity gradient throughout the gap is $-V/R$ and is constant, that is, a straight line (the minus sign merely indicates that the top plate is designated as being at $R = 0$ while the velocity here is $V = V$, and the bottom plate is at $R = R$ while $V = 0$ there). The velocity gradient, which is referred to as the shear rate, has the units of $1/\text{time}$. The force per unit area F/A is known as the shear stress. The velocity and distance can be considered in terms of very small or differential elements, designated as dV and dR, respectively. Then the shear rate becomes $-dV/dR$. A plot can be made of F/A versus $-dV/dR$ or shear stress versus shear rate (see Fig. 2.4). Such a plot characterizes the viscometry of the fluid. The parallel plate system is not a suitable viscometer for blood, since the fluid could not be held in place for measurement. Shear rate ranges and volumes of blood required for commonly used blood viscometers are noted in Table 2.1.

There are two suitable basic viscometric devices that have the analyzable features of the parallel plates and are capable of holding the fluid in place. These viscometers are (a) cone and plate or cone in cone and (b) Couette or narrow-gap concentric cylinder (Fig. 2.5). A guard ring is sometimes employed with a

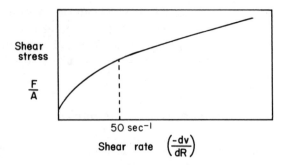

Fig. 2.4   Shear stress F/A versus shear rate dv/dR for blood showing yield stress.

Couette-type viscometer to avoid the effects of denaturation of proteins at the air liquid interface from influencing stress measurement (see Fig. 2.6).

There is some variation of shear rate within a Couette viscometer gap. Although it is possible to obtain exact shear rate calculation using the method of Krieger and Elrod (1953), the use of average shear-rate–shear-stress values across a narrow gap allows determination of the viscometric curve to within a few percentage points of the exact solution (Benis et al., 1971).

Capillary tube viscometers are often used in the measurement of blood viscosity. However, the tube viscometer is not truly a direct measuring viscometer because the flow pattern associated with it is more complex than the characteristic Couette or cone and plate viscometer patterns. Nevertheless, it is inexpensive and capable of great accuracy under the proper conditions.

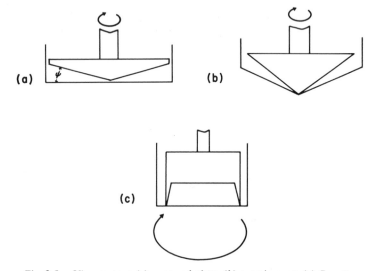

Fig. 2.5   Viscometers: (a) cone and plate, (b) cone in cone, (c) Couette.

Table 2.1   Commonly Used Viscometers for Blood and Plasma

Type	Shear Rate Range for Blood (sec^{-1})	Volume (cm^3)
Brookfield cone and plate LVT	13–230	1.0
Brookfield cone and plate RVT (0.4)[a]	5–1500	0.55
Weissenberg Couette viscometer with cone and plate for end effects and with guard ring	0.001–250	14
GDM Couette viscometer with guard ring	0.001–20	10
Capillary tube viscometer ($D = 500\,\mu$)	0.01–1000	10

[a] This viscometer which has been used extensively in our laboratory has demonstrated excellent precision when properly operated (see Appendix to Chapter 2).

The primary condition is that the flow be uniform or homogeneous throughout the tube; that is, no prominent cell distribution or marginal layer should develop as described in Chapter 3 (see the Appendix to Chapter 2).

Also the flow must be streamline – the Reynolds number for blood $D\bar{V}\rho/K^2$, must be less than 800 (Charm et al., 1968), where D is tube diameter, $\bar{V}$ is mass average velocity, ρ is blood density, and K^2 is "limiting apparent viscosity" for blood.

When these conditions are satisfied, a tube with $D \simeq 500\,\mu$ is usually satisfactory as a viscometer for blood suspensions. In smaller tube diameters, marginal plasma layers may occur with blood flow. It is possible from flow rate and pressure loss information to obtain the wall shear rate τ_w and wall shear stress γ_w.

Wall shear stress in a tube is

$$(2.1) \quad \tau_w = \frac{PD}{4L}$$

where P/L is pressure drop per unit length.

Wall shear rate is

$$(2.2) \quad \gamma_w = 2\frac{\bar{V}}{D}\left[3 + \frac{d\ln(\bar{V}/D)}{d\ln \tau_w}\right]$$

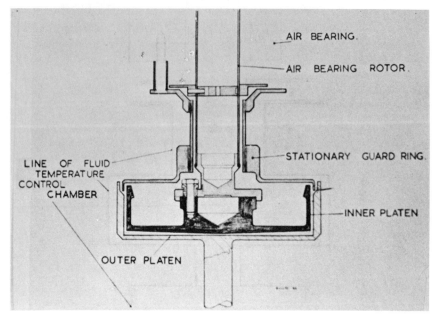

Fig. 2.6 Guard ring on viscometer to prevent influence of surface denaturation on torque measurement of protein suspensions. Outer platen moves, transmitting torque through fluid to inner platen. (Weissenberg Rheogoniometer).

where $(d \ln \overline{V}/D)/(d \ln \tau_w)$ is the slope of $\ln \overline{V}/D$ versus $\ln \tau_w$ (Rabinowitsch, 1929; Mooney, 1931).

The blood flow properties can be evaluated from a plot of τ_w versus γ_w, (e.g., see Fig. 2.7).

In general, Couette or cone and plate viscometers are preferred when they are available because of ease of measurement and the simple analysis of flow in these systems. Detailed discussion of these viscometers can be found in Van Wazer et al. (1963) and Wilkinson (1960); also see the Appendix to Chapter 2.

2.3   SHEAR STRESS – SHEAR RATE RELATIONSHIP OF PLASMA

The shear stress $(\tau = F/A)$ versus shear rate $(\gamma = -dV/dR)$ behavior of plasma is characterized by a straight line passing through the origin (Charm and Kurland, 1962; Copley and Scott-Blair, 1962; Merrill et al., 1964), as indicated in Fig. 2.7. A fluid exhibiting such a plot is known as a Newtonian fluid. The slope of the line is the viscosity. There have also been several reports describing plasma as non-Newtonian (e.g., Gregersen et al., 1965; Cerny et al., 1962; Dintenfass, 1965; Shorthouse and Hutchinson, 1967). For serum and plasma viscosity,

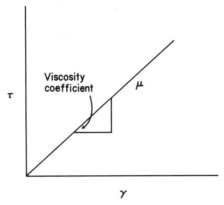

Fig. 2.7 Shear stress versus shear rate diagram for blood plasma. Line follows equation $\tau = \mu\gamma$ where μ is viscosity of plasma.

Bayliss (1952) suggests the relationship $\mu_p/\mu_w = 1/(1 - bc)$, where b is a constant, c is grams of protein per 100 ml, μ_w is water viscosity, and μ_p is plasma viscosity.

Often, when the viscometry plots of plasma measured in cone and plate viscometers down to shear rates of 5 sec^{-1} are extrapolated to zero shear rate, they do not appear to pass through the origin. According to one hypothesis, surface denaturation at the air interface, alluded to previously, causes a protein "skin" to form.

Plasma seldom exhibits this effect in Couette-type viscometers, which have guard rings that prevent the phenomenon described from influencing the measurement. When the measurement of plasma surface layer is excluded by the use of a guard ring on the viscometer, Newtonian flow characteristics are demonstrated. Without a guard ring, plasma displays non-Newtonian behavior (Copley, 1971).

Serum, which has a lower viscosity than plasma due to removal of fibrinogen does not show this deviation from Newtonian behavior in cone and plate viscometers, as plasma sometimes does. This suggests that fibrinogen plays a role in the non-Newtonian behavior of plasma.

Plasma sometimes exhibits time-dependent effects with respect to shear rate. If plasma is subjected to shear rates less than 5 sec^{-1}, the indicated stress will gradually fall to a minimum value. At higher shear rates, the plasma stress achieves the minimum value very rapidly. To observe these changes, care must be taken not to expose the plasma to shear rates greater than 5 sec^{-1} when placing it in the viscometer. The effects are not quickly reversible, if at all, in either case.

These observations suggest that the plasma proteins may form a network throughout the solution which is broken under stress. Attempts to make a direct measurement of strength of this plasma network have been inconclusive thus far. Both the Weissenberg rheogoniometer with Couette attachment and the Brookfield cone and plate viscometer (RVT 0.4) exhibit this time effect. The cone and plate viscometer shows the effect at higher shear rates than the Couette (Charm and Kurland, unpublished data). The initial decrease in plasma viscosity has also been observed in a capillary tube viscometer (shear rate 300 to 500 sec^{-1}) (Scott-Blair, 1970).

Thus we conclude that plasma, particularly at low shear rates, may evidence transitory non-Newtonian behavior which is associated with fibrinogen. This change from non-Newtonian to Newtonian characteristics occurs easily *in vitro* and is not reversible.

The rapid passage of plasma through a narrow hypodermic syringe is sufficient to destroy the non-Newtonian behavior of plasma, suggesting that the non-Newtonian character of plasma perhaps can be maintained *in vivo*.

It has been shown that fibrinogen in plasma subjected to sufficient shear looses its ability to clot (Charm and Wong, 1970). This indicates that plasma does undergo a shear degradation. In fact, the half-life of fibrinogen in the circulation can be explained by shear degradation.

2.4   EFFECT OF TEMPERATURE ON PLASMA VISCOSITY

The Bayliss equation for plasma viscosity noted in Section 2.3 provides for temperature change in the water viscosity term μ_w. Merrill et al. (1963a) have noted that plasma viscosity varies with temperature, as does water when measured with a GDM viscometer. When viscosity is measured in a cone and plate viscometer, however, plasma viscosity does not vary with temperature in the same way as water. The reason for this discrepancy is not known.

A ratio of plasma viscosity to water viscosity as a function of temperature is plotted in Fig. 2.8 (Charm and Kurland, unpublished data). Plasma components have a greater effect on plasma viscosity at 37°C than at 0°C (i.e., plasma viscosity deviates from water viscosity more at 37°C than at 0°C). Proteins and lipids in plasma may be responsible for this difference.

2.5   EFFECT OF PLASMA COMPONENTS ON PLASMA VISCOSITY

The viscosity of plasma increases with its protein concentration, as shown by the Bayliss equation in Section 2.3. However, the various proteins have different influences on plasma viscosity depending on their shape and size. Fibrinogen is the largest of the proteins in plasma, although it forms only 5.5% of plasma

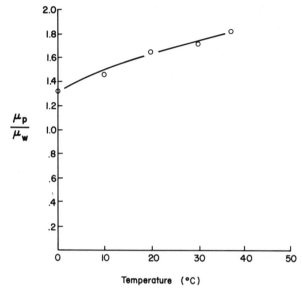

Fig. 2.8 Ratio of plasma viscosity (μ_p) to water viscosity (μ_w) as a function of temperature.

protein. Its influence on plasma viscosity can be seen in the differences between plasma and serum viscosity, serum usually having a viscosity 20% less than plasma.

The effect of globulins (usually 45% of plasma protein) on viscosity is illustrated in the disease macroglobulinemia (Somer, 1966). An increase from 1 to 4 g/100 ml in globulin may cause a 50% increase in plasma viscosity (see Chapter 6).

Albumin, the smallest plasma protein molecule, is present in the largest concentration (approximately 50% of plasma protein). Changes in albumin have the least effect of the three proteins on plasma viscosity, but the substance makes an important contribution to plasma viscosity through its high concentration in plasma.

A high correlation has been found among plasma viscosity, total protein, fibrinogen, and globulins (Mayer, 1966; Rand et al., 1970). High albumin concentrations in plasma are accompanied at times by reduced globulin concentrations, actually resulting in lowered plasma viscosities. It has also been suggested that albumin may "neutralize" the viscosity effect of other proteins in plasma (Mayer, 1966).

When plasma viscosity is elevated in disease (Chapter 6), it is mostly accompanied by increased α globulin, and fibrinogen concentrations (Kogai et al., 1971). Beta lipoprotein and lipalbumin have little effect on plasma viscosity.

It is clear that fibrinogen and globulin concentrations have the greatest influence on blood plasma viscosity.

2.6   SHEAR STRESS – SHEAR RATE CHARACTERISTICS OF RED CELL SUSPENSION

Suspension of cells in plasma up to a volume fraction ϕ of 0.05 have a steady shear-stress–shear-rate relationship typical of Newtonian fluid. The viscosity of such suspensions when ϕ is less than 0.05 is expressed with reasonable accuracy by Einstein's equation for spheres in suspension (Einstein, 1906, Jeffery, 1922).

$$(2.3) \quad \mu_s = \mu_p \frac{1}{1 - \alpha\phi}$$

where μ_p = plasma viscosity

μ_s = suspension viscosity

α = shape factor (2.5 for spheres)

The constant 2.5 theoretically varies with the shape of the particle, but it appears to apply to red cells when ϕ is less than 0.05. The volume fraction includes not only the volume fraction of the particles but the volume fraction of the particles plus absorbed fluid, as well.

One of the assumptions underlying equation 2.3 is that the particles behave as individuals and do not interact significantly.

As ϕ increases from 0.05, the suspension viscosity varies from equation 2.3 because the interaction between particles becomes more significant and the properties associated with the interaction (e.g., cell elasticity, aggregation, eddy flow) now influence viscosity. Eddy flow refers to the streamline flow patterns around cells or aggregates.

Over the years, many empirical equations have been suggested to express blood viscosity as a function of cell concentration and plasma viscosity (e.g., Bayliss, 1952). These relations generally take the form of equation 2.3. Thus we have the Hatschek (1920) equation, determined for emulsions with tightly packed, flat polyhedra droplets

$$\frac{\mu_s}{\mu_p} = \frac{1}{1 - \phi^{1/3}}$$

or the expression due to Jeffery (1922)

$$\frac{\mu_s}{\mu_p} = \frac{1 + \phi}{1 - b\phi}$$

where b is a constant depending on shape of the particle.

Cokelet (1963a) has suggested that for red cell suspensions

$$(2.4) \quad \frac{\mu_s}{\mu_p} = \frac{1}{(1 - \phi)^{2.5}}$$

With a cone and plate viscometer, the limiting apparent viscosity of red cell suspensions is found to be correlated up to $\phi = 0.6$ by equation 2.3, in which α is expressed by

$$(2.5) \quad \alpha = 0.070 \exp\left(2.49\phi + \frac{1107}{T} \exp -1.69\phi\right)$$

where T is absolute temperature (°K), that is, 273+°C (Charm and Kurland, unpublished).

A plot of α against ϕ for $T = 25°C$ and $37°C$ is presented in Fig. 2.9.

Other equations similar in form to equation 2.3 have been proposed (e.g., Bingham and White, 1911; Hess, 1920):

$$\frac{\mu_s}{\mu_p} = \frac{1}{1 - \phi}$$

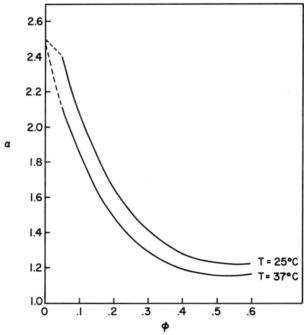

Fig. 2.9 α versus ϕ (for calculation of suspension viscosity up to $\phi = 0.6$), see equation (2.5).

Nubar (1967)

$$\frac{\mu_a}{\mu_p} = \frac{\lambda}{\lambda - \phi}$$

where λ is concentration of packed cells = 0.75 (a constant).

Figure 2.10 compares these equations, and it is clear that there is little agreement between them (Nubar, 1967) and that none is satisfactory for estimating limiting "apparent" blood viscosities above $\phi = 0.6$.

Since α varies with temperature (equation 2.5), it may be that the number of cell interactions per unit time changes with temperature; alternatively the energy loss per collision may change. It is possible that the elasticity of the cells varies with temperature, thus causing change in momentum and energy loss upon collision. A temperature-related change in the internal viscosity of the cell may influence cell elasticity, hence suspension viscosity. Bayliss (1952) notes that the effect of temperature on blood viscosity can be estimated from

$$\frac{(\mu_s/\mu_w)_T}{(\mu_s/\mu_w)_{T+20}} = 1.09$$

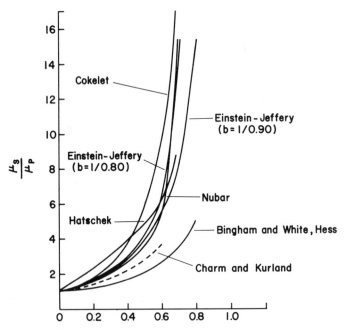

Fig. 2.10   Calculated relative apparent viscosity versus cell volume fraction from various equations (adapted from Nubar, 1967). Charm and Kurland calculation from equations 2.3 and 2.5.

However, this assumes that the relative viscosity of plasma does not vary with temperature, which has not been established (see Fig. 2.8). Rat blood relative viscosity does not vary with temperature (Shorrock and Hillman, 1969).

Merrill et al. (1963a), using a GDM Couette viscometer, tested the relative viscosity of blood to water between 10 and 37°C and found it to be independent of temperature at shear rates above 1 sec^{-1}. This is clearly in disagreement with equations 2.3 and 2.5, but in agreement with equation 2.4 and the equations of Nubar, Hess, and Hatschek. Equation 2.3 with equation 2.5 has been tested with a cone and plate viscometer and found to be in agreement within 10%; see Table 2.2.

Table 2.2   A Comparison of Experimental and Calculated Values of Blood Viscosity Using Equations 2.3 and 2.5

ϕ	μ_p (P)	α^a	$\mu_{s\,exp}$ (P)	$\mu_{s\,calc}$ (P)	$T(°C)$
0.590	0.0144	1.25	0.0557	0.0553	25
0.430	0.0144	1.28	0.0324	0.0320	25
0.430	0.0169	1.28	0.0375	0.0375	25
0.400	0.0149	1.30	0.0404	0.0310	25
0.448	0.0156	1.27	0.0368	0.0361	25
0.418	0.0152	1.28	0.0350	0.0330	25
0.458	0.0144	1.27	0.0396	0.0348	25
0.461	0.0199	1.26	0.0272	0.0268	37
0.427	0.0131	1.23	0.0289	0.0272	37
0.460	0.0115	1.21	0.0272	0.0258	37
0.400	0.0110	1.23	0.0262	0.0210	37
0.361	0.0110	1.25	0.0193	0.0200	37

[a]From 0.070 exp (2.49 ϕ + 1107/T exp -1.61 ϕ) = α, where T = °K

Barbee (1973) notes that at shear rates greater than 1 sec^{-1}, the viscosity of blood relative to the viscosity of plasma is independent of temperature and the type of viscometer used. Below 1 sec^{-1}, however, the relative viscosity of blood decreases as temperature increases. Barbee suggests that shear rate, shear stress gradients, and flexibility are important aspects of temperature dependence of whole blood relative viscosity in a capillary viscometer.

The internal viscosity of a red cell was claculated using a modification of Taylor's equation for the viscosity of dilute emulsions (Dintenfass, 1971):

$$\mu_r = \frac{1}{(1 - \phi T)^{2.5}}$$

where μ_r = relative viscosity of blood to plasma

$$T = (P + 0.4)/(P + 1)$$

$$P = \mu_i/\mu_p$$

μ_i = internal viscosity of cell

μ_p = plasma viscosity

When blood viscosity is measured at shear rates high enough to prevent aggregation, the internal viscosity of red cells in isotonic solutions is 0.029 P (Dintenfass, 1971).

The Dintenfass equation for blood viscosity can be compared with experimental values. When μ_p = 0.0144 P and ϕ = 0.59, the experimental cone and plate blood viscosity is 0.0577 P at 25°C. If μ_i = 0.029 P, then T = 0.8, and blood viscosity by the Dintenfass equation is 0.069 P. Using equation 2.3, this value is 0.0533 P.

In another case when ϕ = 0.418, μ_p = 0.0152 P, and blood viscosity is experimentally 0.0350 P, it is calculated by the Dintenfass equation to be 0.041 P. From equation 2.3 it is found to be 0.0330 P.

In summary, temperature may affect the viscosity of blood through:

1. Plasma viscosity.
2. Red cell wall elasticity.
3. Viscosity of cell contents.
4. Cell shape.

2.7   POWER LAW EXPRESSIONS FOR BLOOD VISCOSITY

Some investigators (e.g., Charm and Kurland, 1962; Hershey et al., 1966) have suggested a power law expression as a means of characterizing blood viscosity:

(2.6) $\tau = b\gamma^s$

where b and s are constants.

It has been found that this form of the equation does not hold over more than two decades of shear rates with constant values of b and s (Charm et al., 1965).

Therefore, flow constants determined from equation 2.6 have limited use for application to flow analysis in capillary tubes or vessels unless shear rates in the tube are definitely within the experimental range measured with the viscometer.

2.8   HERSCHEL–BULKLEY EQUATION

The Herschel-Bulkley equation (Herschel and Bulkley, 1926), which follows, has a realistic physical basis (Scott-Blair, 1967).

(2.7) $\tau = b\gamma^s + C$

where C is the blood yield stress or shear strength.

This expression is derived by relating the stress required to break interparticle bonds and the number of bonds at any time on the assumption that doubling γ would halve the number of bonds that could re-form.

However, equation 2.7 does not fit the flow-rate–stress relationship for blood over a wide range of shear rates (Charm et al., 1965). The methods for determining the yield stress are discussed later.

2.9   CASSON EQUATION FOR BLOOD VISCOSITY

Casson (1958) derived a semiempirical equation to describe the flow behavior of printing ink, and Reiner and Scott-Blair (1959) suggested its application to describe blood viscosity:

(2.8) $\tau^{1/2} = K\gamma^{1/2} + C^{1/2}$

where C = yield stress or shear strength of the suspension determined by extrapolation from above 1 sec^{-1}

K = Casson "viscosity"

Casson's equation is based on the behavior of mutually attractive particles subjected to disruptive forces such that particle group size is a function of shear rate. In addition, the yield stress or shear strength of the suspension must be exceeded before the structure can be broken and flow initiated.

It has been shown that the shear-stress–shear-rate behavior of red cell suspensions can be expressed by this equation over a wide range of cell concentrations and shear rates (1 to 100,000 sec^{-1}) (Charm and Kurland, 1962, 1965) and 0.1 to 20 sec^{-1} (Merrill et al., 1964; Cokelet et al., 1963b).

Summary of Equations Describing Blood Shear Stress–Shear Rate Behavior

Neither the power law expression nor the Herschel-Bulkley equation can be used to express blood flow properties over more than two decades. The Herschel-Bulkley equation has the added disadvantage of requiring three constants, whereas power law or Casson equations require only two.

One approach to generalizing the Herschel-Bulkley and Casson equations assumes that bonds between particles are gradually broken with increase in shear rate (Oka, 1971). This results in a fundamental differential equation to determine flow curves of non-Newtonian suspensions:

$$\frac{d\tau}{(T + C)^a} = K\frac{d\gamma}{(\gamma + \beta)^a}$$

where α, C, K, β are constants.

When a is 1, the Herschel-Bulkley equation results; when a is $\frac{1}{2}$, the Casson equation results.

The Casson equation appears to be the best for expressing the relationships of τ and γ for normal blood from the range of shear rates in which the yield stress effects are prominent through the high shear rates where yield stress effects are negligible. Below 1 sec^{-1}, shear stress data does not always follow Casson's equation as closely as above 1 sec^{-1} (Merrill et al., 1966), but this discrepancy may be due to artifacts in low shear rate viscometry.

2.10   CASSON VISCOSITY K AND LIMITING APPARENT VISCOSITY K^2

When the yield stress is very small compared with the shear stress, equation 2.8 reduces to that for a Newtonian fluid and K^2 becomes the limiting apparent viscosity or the equivalent of μ_s in equation 2.3. Thus we have

$$(2.9) \quad K^2 = \frac{\mu_p}{1 - \alpha\phi}$$

where α is defined by equation 2.5.

Also from equation 2.8 we can write

$$(2.10) \quad \tau - 2\tau^{1/2}C^{1/2} + C = K^2\gamma$$

and

$$\frac{\tau}{\gamma} = K^2 + 2\frac{\tau^{1/2}C^{1/2}}{\gamma} - \frac{C}{\gamma} = \text{apparent viscosity.}$$

It can be seen that when the terms involving C are small compared with K^2, the apparent viscosity τ/γ is constant and is equal to K^2. These terms become smaller as shear rate γ increases. When γ is small, the terms become large compared with K^2, and the apparent viscosity increases. Thus the change in apparent viscosity with shear rate is due to the yield stress associated with the aggregation of cells and to change in cell shape. An example of this is shown in Fig. 2.11. When yield stress effects are absent, the suspension shear-stress—shear-rate relationship becomes that of a Newtonian fluid.

The term K^2 varies with temperature and concentration according to equation 2.9, where α has the relationship indicated in equation 2.5 or Fig. 2.9.

Another problem in the measurement of Casson viscosity in blood arises because measurements with Couette viscometers and cone and plate viscometers do not agree. The value of K^2 is 10 to 20% less by cone and plate viscometry than with Couette viscometry. The reason for this is not known for certain (Charm and Kurland 1968a). Since plasma viscosities are the same in these two viscometers, the effect must be associated with different cell distributions in these devices.

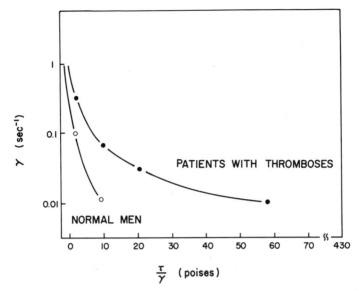

Fig. 2.11   Shear rate vs apparent blood viscosity (adapted from Dintenfass, 1966). As shear rate increases apparent viscosity, τ/γ, approaches limiting value.

2.11   BLOOD YIELD STRESS

The yield stress or shear strength of blood is determined by the cell-to-cell contact and by the cell aggregate structure (see Fig. 2.1). It is difficult to measure yield stress because of the interaction of the measuring instruments with the red cell structure. Little is actually understood of the detailed instrument–cell-structure contact, and it is questionable whether most direct measurements of blood yield stress are measurements of the blood structure or of the structure–instrument interface.

There are five principal methods employed for the measurement of yield stress. These are given below.

Extrapolation of $\tau^{1/2}$ versus $\gamma^{1/2}$ Plot to Zero Shear Rate

The intercept in the $\tau^{1/2}$ versus $\gamma^{1/2}$ extrapolation is the square root of the yield stress (see equation 2.8 and Fig. 2.12. Yield stresses obtained by extrapolation from 0.1 sec^{-1} to zero often do not agree with extrapolation from 1 sec^{-1}. A 50% difference in yield stress may be expected between these two extrapolation methods (Cokelet et al., 1963; Merrill et al., 1966).

At finite shear rates, the shear stress is associated with suspension movement as well as the yield stress effect. In extrapolating to zero shear rate, it is assumed

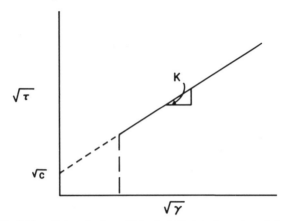

Fig. 2.12   Determination of blood yield stress by extrapolation.

that the relative effect of fluid motion on shear stress remains constant. Hence experiments with clay suspensions indicate that yield stress depends on the shear pattern in the fluid (Boardman and Whitmore, 1961).

At low shear rates the suspension may not remain uniform in the viscometer; rather, two phases may develop with a fluid phase at the instrument interface. It has been observed that when very low shear rates (e.g., 0.01 sec^{-1}) are present in blood, the $\tau^{1/2}$ versus $\gamma^{1/2}$ curve extrapolates to $\tau^{1/2}$ equals zero (i.e., no yield stress is evident). The effect, which has also been observed in a Weissenberg Couette viscometer, has been attributed to the development of a plasma layer at the moving surface (Chien et al., 1966).

A marginal plasma layer has been observed in a GDM Couette viscometer (Cokelet, 1963). It has been proposed that the surfaces of the GDM viscometer be ruled with fine grooves to prevent the formation of two phases, but this measure does not appear to help.

At low shear rates (below 10 sec^{-1}), it has been shown that the cells in a cone and plate viscometer aggregate "squeezing out" the plasma (Schmid-Schönbein et al., 1968). All this points to the possibility of artifacts associated with low shear rate viscometry which can affect the determination of yield stress by extrapolation. To distinguish between yield stresses found from high shear rate (i.e., above 1 sec^{-1}) and low shear rate extrapolation, we use C (applicable to high shear rate) and τ_y (low or zero shear rate).

Torque Decay Method

The torque decay method is a direct measurement of blood yield stress (Merrill et al., 1965a). The blood sample in the viscometer is stressed and allowed to come to rest. The residual torque at rest measures the yield stress. However, the torque reaches zero after some time and it is essential that the appropriate time for measurement be selected (i.e., when the residual torque has developed and the cell structure is still intact). Good agreement has been reported between this method and the low shear rate extrapolation method (Merrill et al., 1965a).

From measurements in a Weissenberg rheogoniometer between shear rates of 10^{-3} to 10^3 sec^{-1}, a discontinuity occurs between 10^{-1} and 10^{-2} sec^{-1} which is attributed to the yield stress (Copley et al., 1973). The torque at the discontinuity is in close agreement with the residual yield value from the recorded relaxation curve after rotation has stopped.

Pressure Decay Method

In principle the pressure decay method is similar to the torque decay approach except that a capillary tube viscometer is used together with a pressure transducer to measure the residual pressure after flow has stopped in a capillary tube (Merrill et al., 1965a). Pressure decay is subject to the same problems as the torque decay method, since the residual pressure may rapidly diminish to zero because of structure breakdown or syneresis at the instrument wall. However, good agreement is reported between this method, the extrapolation method, and torque decay method. In practice, pressure decay systems are much more difficult to operate than torque decay systems.

Balance Plate Method

A plate immersed in a blood sample is attached to a sensitive balance. After gentle oscillation, the plate is allowed to come to rest, and the residual force acting on the plate is measured and related to the yield stress. Measurements of yield stress by this method give lower values than the torque or extrapolation methods (Benis and Lacoste, 1968). For whole blood, yield stresses from Couette viscometry range from 0.015 to 0.05 dyne/cm^2, whereas from the balance plate method the values are between 0.002 and 0.008 dyne/cm^2.

The repeatability of yield stress measurements by the plate method is 20 to 50%. This lack of precision in yield stress measurements is thought to be due to the nonhomogeneity of blood (Benis and Lacoste 1968).

Sedimentation in Tapered Tube

The sedimentation method for determining yield stress depends on finding the tube diameter that just supports a column of structured cells and prevents settling (Charm and Kurland, 1967). Like all the methods discussed except extrapolation, it assumes that the bonding between instrument and cells is stronger than that between cells.

In this method a microhematocrit tube is drawn to a taper and the blood sample is admitted through capillary action. The tube is taped to a microscope slide and held vertically for a few moments until the column of cells breaks. The diameter at the point of breaking (yield diameter) is measured with a low-power microscope (see Figs. 2.13 and 2.14). The yield diameter is related to the yield stress in a tube with a small taper angle by

$$(2.11) \quad \tau_y = \frac{(g)(\phi)(\rho_c - \rho_p)D_y}{4 \cos \phi}$$

where τ_y = yield stress, (determined from shear rates below 1 sec^{-1}; in this case at zero sec^{-1}

g = gravitational constant, 980.8 cm/sec^2

ρ_c = density of cells

ρ_p = density of plasma (cell and plasma density must be measured using a copper sulfate technique — Wintrobe (1962)

D_y = diameter at point of break (cm)

ϕ = taper angle (cos $\phi \cong 1$ for small angles)

In this case, it is possible to observe the cell—wall relationships at the time the cell column breaks. There may be considerable disturbance in this region before rupture of the column is complete (Fig. 2.14).

Sedimentation is the only method that permits direct observation of the cell structure as measurement is made. The time before the structure disintegrates completely varies considerably. It is questionable whether one is measuring the strength of the cell—cell structure or of the cell—wall structure. Values of blood

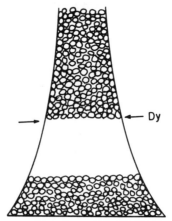

Fig. 2.13   Yield diameter in settling red cell suspension.

yield stress for this method are in the range of 0.1 to 0.30 dyne/cm^2 and are generally in agreement with extrapolation of shear stress from above 1 sec^{-1} for data taken with a cone and plate viscometer. Agreement does not appear, however, with data from Couette viscometers or with values measured by balance plate or torque decay method (differences between cone and plate and Couette blood viscometry were noted previously).

Summary of Yield Stress Measurement Methods

The yield stress of blood ranges from 0.003 to 0.20 dyne/cm^2, depending on which method is employed for measurement. The extrapolation method using $\tau^{1/2}$ versus $\gamma^{1/2}$ is probably the most nearly correct, although artifacts may occur with measurements at low shear rates (below 1 sec^{-1}). Extrapolation from high shear rates has less precision because of the greater extrapolation, but this approach avoids such low shear rate artifacts. There is no agreement about which method is the most accurate.

The problem in understanding yield stress and the effect of cell volume fraction may be clarified by an analysis of blood yield stress for a hypothetical blood suspension between two parallel plates (see Fig. 2.15). Assume that there is no slippage at the wall and that the structure, when it yields, is broken in the plane of the dotted line with an area A and not at the wall. Cells cannot

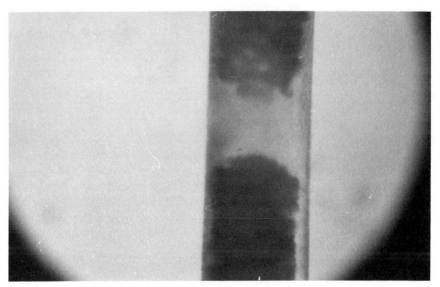

Fig. 2.14   Blood suspension breaking at "yield diameter" in section of vertical tapered tube (x100); note gap at wall in settling section.

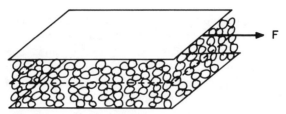

Fig. 2.15   Red cell suspension in hypothetical parallel plate viscometer. Doubling the cell concentration doubles the contact area in the plane of shear.

contribute to the shear strength of the cell network unless they somehow increase the shear resistance of the structure. Given the structure of cells formed between the two plates of a hypothetical viscometer, it is obvious from the random distribution of rouleaux that some cells or rouleaux do not contribute to increasing the shear strength of the structure. In an idealized case, however, the maximum shear strength would be realized if all rouleaux were formed into columns bridging the space between the two plates and if shear force exerted by moving one of the plates were distributed among the cross sections of all the rouleau columns.

If the dimensions of the space between the plates are x, y, and z, where z is the distance between plates, the total number of cells in the space between plates is $N = \phi xyz/N_0$, where N_0 is the number of cells per column. In a column, the cells are stacked on their "flat" side, which has an average thickness t_c. Thus $N_0 = z/t_c$, and the number of columns is $N_c = \phi xyt_c$. The surface area over which the shear force acts in this ideal case is the $N_c \times$ cross-sectional area of a column, or πr_c^2, where r_c is the cell radius. The surface over which the shear force must act in breaking the cell structure is then $\pi \phi xyt_c r_c^2$.

The shear strength of each column is constant. The force required to shear the cell structure F_s is proportional to the number of rouleau columns and their associated area, which is, in this ideal case, proportional to ϕ, the cell volume fraction. Since the yield stress is F_s/xy, the yield stress is also proportional to ϕ.

It is possible that all cells do not contribute to the strength of the structure. The size and number of rouleaux that form are a function of the number of cell collisions that occur, having the correct orientation and appropriate energy level. Again, this number will be directly proportional to the cell concentration if the cell interaction to form rouleaux is considered on a model of a chemical reaction. Even in the nonideal case (where all cells do not contribute to the shear strength of the suspension), it appears that the yield stress is directly proportional to or a linear function of the cell concentration.

This analysis clearly suggests that the true yield stress should be a linear function of cell concentration. However, this model does not consider a complex pattern of cell interaction and packing with cross linking between columns of cells.

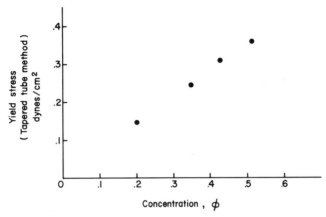

Fig. 2.16   Variation of yield stress by tapered tube method as function of cell volume fraction (25°C).

The settling tube method for yield stress does result in a linear relationship between yield stress and cell volume fraction (see Fig. 2.16). Using extrapolation from low shear rate data, however, yield stress is found to be a square function of cell concentration (Merrill et al., 1965b). Again, it is uncertain which is correct.

In another theoretical approach, Seaman (1967) computed the force necessary to separate red cells by application of the Derjaquin-Landau-Verwey-Overbeek theory for a spherical model. He considered the net force arising from the electrostatic repulsion and long-range London-van der Waals attractive forces between individual cells. From his calculations, the force to separate cells is in the order of 0.1 dyne/cm^2. This is the order of range of blood yield stress. However, as pointed out in theoretical analysis, yield stress is a function of factors other than the force binding cells together.

2.12   EFFECT OF RED CELL FLEXIBILITY ON VISCOSITY

It has been suggested that cell flexibility influences blood viscosity, particularly at high hematocrit values. Thus suspensions of the cells made inelastic with acetaldehyde exhibit Newtonian properties at low shear rates, whereas normal cells do not (Chien et al., 1967). At high shear rates (about 50 sec^{-1}), moreover, hardened cells show a "shear thickening" effect and normal cells exhibit "shear thinning" behavior (Chien et al., 1969; Dintenfass, 1965; Chien et al., 1970).

Cell rigidity is related to the characteristics of the cell contents as well as the cell membrane. The cell membrane is capable of moving around the cell contents, much as a tank tread would move around the wheels

(Schmid-Schönbein and Wells, 1971a). The evidence for this lies in the viscosity of packed cells, which is much lower than would be expected (Dintenfass, 1968a). In this case, the viscosity of the cell contents (e.g., hemoglobin) is the controlling viscosity factor.

The shear deformation of red cells is a function of the viscosity ratio between external medium and intracellular hemoglobin fluid. The deformability of red cells is a major cause of the decrease in blood viscosity at high shear rates (Usami and Chien, 1972). Cells deform into prolate ellipsoids, and the membrane rotates around the cell contents at shear stresses of 5 dynes/cm^2 and above. Schmid-Schönbein et al. (1971a) demonstrated that the deformation increases with increasing shear rate as shown by the Rumscheidt equation (Rumscheidt and Mason, 1961):

$$(2.12) \quad D = \frac{L - B}{L + B} = \frac{\gamma r_c \mu_p}{\sigma} \frac{(19\mu_p/\mu_i) + 16}{(16\mu_p/\mu_i) + 16}$$

where γ = rate of shear
   L = length
   B = breadth of ellipsoid
   μ_p = viscosity of continuous medium
   μ_i = internal viscosity
   σ = interfacial tension (plasma-RBC)
   r_c = cell radius

The internal viscosity of red cells has been calculated to range between 1 and 6 centipoises (cP) (Dintenfass 1968a, 1968b). This estimate includes cell membrane effects as well as hemoglobin viscosity.

Movement of the cell membrane around the cell contents is the mechanism by which red cells adapt themselves to flow. Hemoglobin is subjected to shear, the cell assumes the properties of a fluid drop, and whole blood behaves as an emulsion rather than as a suspension.

The viscoelastic properties of the erythrocyte membrane result in both stress and time thresholds relating hemoglobin release to both the magnitude and the duration of the applied shear stress (Williams, 1972).

Rosenblum and Warren (1973) have noted a rise in blood viscosity in a GDM Couette viscometer, apparently due to cell damage after 10 min of shearing. Refrigeration prior to shearing precluded the effect.

Deformability in pathological states may be reduced because of either membrane defects or hemoglobin abnormality. Abnormal molecular interactions with reciprocal binding of cellular constituents represent the basic mechanism responsible for increased red cell rigidity. Intracellular glutathione reduces the interactions and is the primary protective agent against loss of cell deformability. A lowered intracellular ATP level allows the formation of calcium bridges between cell constituents, thus causing increased cell rigidity (Teitel, 1971), and it has been shown that fresh red cells are more flexible than stored cells (Sirs, 1968). The higher viscosity associated with old stored cells might be influenced by the increased rigidity of the older cells (Usami et al., 1971). This relationship may be associated with change in the charge on older cells, but the effect of surface charges on cell deformability is not defined (Danon et al., 1969).

The viscosity of sickle cells, which have lost filtrability, with a 34% hematocrit is almost identical to a normal control of 45% (Schmid-Schönbein, 1971).

Osmotic pressure also influences cell deformability, either by changing internal viscosity of hemoglobin or making the cell membrane more rigid.

Surfactants appear to affect cell rigidity and to influence viscosity. Sodium oleate lowered blood viscosity in concentrations of 20 to 40 mg%, but at 60 mg% it caused membrane stiffening, thus raising the viscosity (Ehrley, 1968). Not only does cell deformability affect viscosity directly, but it may also affect plasma flow patterns between cells and their boundary layers. The flow of a rigid cell model past a stationary one has a marked effect on fluid energy loss (Bugliarello et al., 1969a).

None of the equations presented previously for estimating blood viscosity at high shear rates has included a term for cell rigidity. These empirical equations were determined with normal blood where the influence of cell deformability is relatively constant. However, diseased states that affect cell flexibility would cause substantial errors in estimating blood viscosity, for example, using equation 2.3. Cell flexibility influences blood flow primarily through the value of α.

2.13 MEASUREMENT OF CELL FLEXIBILITY

Cell deformability has been measured by three methods.

1. Viscometry of packed red cell mass.
2. Rate of packing of red cell column during centrifugation.
3. Passage through polycarbonate sieves.

All these methods are indirect and difficult to analyze; moreover, they are influenced by factors other than those involved with flexibility. For example, the amount of plasma trapped between cells interferes with the measurement of flexibility by viscometric methods (Jacobs, 1963; Thomas and Janes, 1966; Johnson, 1969).

In the centrifugal packing method, the compression of cells during centrifugation is due to the weight of the packed cells pressing down on one another. As trapped plasma is completely eliminated between the cells, an increase can be observed in the density of the column and consequently in the total pressure acting on the cells. Since, however, osmotic action would immediately release water into the extracellular space, the compression force is determined by a number of factors – height of cell column, density difference between cells and plasma, centrifugal force, and time applied (Sirs, 1968). A centrifugally packed column of hardened cells appears to contain only 60% of the plasma as compared with 100% for normal cells due to distribution of plasma, (Chien, et al., 1968).

Cell deformability measurement by passage through polycarbonate sieves probably lends itself to analysis more readily than other methods. Increases in the viscosity of cells hardened by acetaldehyde occur within 2 to 3 hours, but no change in flexibility is observed by the centrifugal packing method or passage through sieves for 12 hours (Chien et al., 1971a). These findings suggest that the viscometric method may be the most sensitive.

2.14 PLASMA FACTORS AFFECTING BLOOD FLOW PROPERTIES

Aggregation of red cells is reflected in the yield stress. The cell aggregating capacity of plasma increases with increasing protein concentration, and it has been suggested that fibrinogen is the principal plasma protein affecting cell aggregation (Merrill, et al., 1963c). Fibrinogen shows a specific aggregating activity 19 times higher than that of normal plasma (Hint and Arfors, 1971), and the flow properties of blood are improved by destroying fibrinogen with streptokinase (Ehrly, 1971). Fibrinogen added to cells has less aggregating effect than does native fibrinogen, and type A cells are affected more than type O cells.

It has been proposed that the aggregating effect of fibrinogen is caused by the fibrinogen molecule being absorbed "end on" into craterlike sites on the surface of the cell at one of its terminal ball-shaped elements; the other terminal ball of the molecule is projected outward for subsequent engagement with an absorbing site on the membrane of neighboring cell (Merrill et al., 1966).

Merrill et al. (1965b) observed that fibrinogen added to cells in saline solution also produces increased aggregation and suggested an equation for calculating τ_y (the yield stress determined at shear rates below 1 sec^{-1}).

$$(2.13) \quad \tau_y^{1/2} = 0.36B \left(\frac{1}{1-\phi} - 1 \right)$$

where B is the function of fibrinogen concentration (see Table 2.3).

Equation 2.13, which applies up to $\phi = 0.80$ (Chien et al., 1966), agrees with yield stress values determined in a GDM Couette viscometer but not with cone and plate viscometer data.

Yield stress by the tapered tube method varies linearly with hematocrit (see Fig. 2.16, which indicates the yield diameter D_y in equation 2.11 remains constant).

Table 2.3 B as a Function of Fibrinogen Concentration[a]

B	Fibrinogen (g/100 ml of plasma + ACD solution)
0.894	0.21
0.875	0.21
0.940	0.24
0.930	0.24
1.01	0.27
1.05	0.28
1.10	0.35
1.09	8.36
1.18	0.46

[a] From Merrill et al. (1956b).

Red cells in serum (i.e., with no fibrinogen present) also possess a yield stress when measured in a GDM viscometer (Chien et al., 1966), although in this case it is about half that measured for cells in plasma. Merrill et al. (1965b) found no yield stress in serum. Minute amounts of fibrinogen—fribin complexes lead to a dramatic increase in yield stress (Copley et al., 1967). At sufficiently high concentrations, cells in saline possess a yield stress – about one quarter that of cells in plasma (Chien et al., 1966). Red cells also aggregate or display a yield stress in the absence of fibrinogen when in pathological sera (Wells et al., 1971).

Wells (1965) used a GDM viscometer to investigate the effects of plasma albumin, fibrinogen, and globulin on blood viscosity between shear rates of 0.1 and 20 sec^{-1}. He noted that albumin tends to decrease cell aggregation, possibly because of its strong negative charge. Fibrinogen, which has a slightly negative charge in plasma and is a much longer molecule than albumin, has the greatest influence in promoting cell aggregation. Globulin also produces cell aggregation, but not as strongly as fibrinogen. Although red cells aggregate easily into rouleau forms in solutions of fibrinogen, the sedimentation of these aggregates is not rapid until the normal physiological concentration (0.2 to 0.5 g%) is exceeded.

The importance of factors other than fibrinogen has been further investigated by Wells et al. (1971). Using torque decay methods, cell aggregation and finite yield stress were found with pathological sera which had clottable proteins removed. Globulin had the most profound effect on blood viscosity, and albumin the least effect. When flow in the bulbar conjunctiva is examined directly, it is found that the relation between plasma protein levels and cell aggregation *in vivo* is considerably less predictable than that of red cell suspensions *in vitro*.

There are species differences in the hemorheological effects of serum globulins. For example, the elephant has a higher concentration of β_2 globulin which may be similar to firbinogen in its ability to cause rouleau formation (Chien et al., 1971b). Other plasma proteins in saline have about the same effect on cells as does saline (i.e., cell aggregation is minimal) (Merrill et al., 1966).

Red cell aggregation can be produced by gelatin, high molecular weight dextran (greater than 60,000) but not low molecular weight dextran. Factors changing the normal shape and deformability hinder aggregate formation. Lowering the salinity of red cell suspensions in plasma or serum first produces decreasing aggregate formation until, at a conductivity below 1 ms a sharp increase of red cell aggregate and clump formation takes place. Red cells in isotonic solutions of albumin or dextran 40 at normal salinity (5 mhos at $\phi = 0.45$) do not show any aggregation.

Bovine blood, incapable of aggregate formation in normal plasma, also does form aggregates when the salinity is reduced below 0.5 mhos. Here, however, the aggregation is weaker than in human blood under identical conditions. It is suggested that red cell aggregation is not caused by a specific binding process of distinct proteins but is rather the consequence of a nonspecific adhesive plasma protein of minimum molecular weight and the cell surface (Volger et al., 1972).

2.15   EFFECTS OF OSMOTIC PRESSURE ON BLOOD VISCOSITY

Both cell elasticity and cell shape influence blood viscosity. The osmotic pressure difference across a red cell membrane determines to a large extent its shape, size, and elasticity. Therefore, it is not surprising to find that changes in osmotic pressure cause changes in blood viscosity.

The $\tau-\gamma$ relationship of red cells in hypotonic and hypertonic solutions was measured using a GDM viscometer (Meiselman et al., 1967). In solutions having equal numbers of red cells, the yield stress of the suspension increased and viscosity decreased as the solution varied from hypertonic to hypotonic. Although the number of red cells remained constant, the hematocrit varied from 34.8% at 381 mosm/kg to 42.7% at 276 mosm/kg. The increase in yield stress with increasing hematocrit could be expected, but not the decrease in viscosity with increasing hematocrit.

In a study of the mechanical properties of red cells, the erythrocyte membrane in 1.2% NaCl solution (hypertonic) exhibited less resistance to deformation and only slight resistance to bending (Rand and Burton, 1964). However, cells in isotonic or hypotonic saline (0.6% NaCl) appear to be identical in membrane properties, being much more rigid than those in hypertonic saline.

From these observations, it seems that a hypotonic red cell suspension should have a lower apparent viscosity than either an isotonic or hypotonic suspension. This contradicts the results of Meiselman et al. (1967), who suggest that the differences are due to the removal of proteins and lipoproteins from saline-washed membranes, which would also affect membrane characteristics.

The red cell sedimentation rate is increased in hypotonic solutions. This effect may be due to the increased tendency of red cells to aggregate, as shown by the increased yield stress in hypotonic solutions mentioned previously.

The variation in cell volume with tonicity is given by Ponder (1940) as

$$(2.14) \quad \frac{V_c}{V_{iso}} = RW \left(\frac{1}{T} - 1 \right) + 1$$

where V_c = new volume of cells
V_{iso} = volume of cells in an isotonic medium
W = volume fraction of water in cells, generally 0.7
T = ratio of osmolarity of medium to that of an isotonic (0.9%) NaCl solution
R = correction factor for nonideal osmotic behavior of the solute — generally, R varies from 0.9 to 1.02

In Meiselman's study, for the same number of red cells, the hematocrit (H) varies with tonicity as follows:

276 mosm/kg $H = 42.7$
300 mosm/kg $H = 40.1$
329 mosm/kg $H = 38.0$
381 mosm/kg $H = 34.2$

Using equation 2.14 with $R = 1$ and with 276 mosm/kg, $H = 42.7$ as a standard, it is calculated that $H = 40.1$ for 300 mosm/kg and $H = 34.2$ for 381 mosm/kg.

Thus Ponder's equation closely agrees with Meiselman's data and is suitable for predicting cell volume changes as a function of tonicity, which in turn influences viscosity and yield stress changes as described previously.

Packed cells from hypotonic saline show a greater viscosity than normal packed cells, but crenated packed cells from hypertonic solutions display a still greater viscosity than either normal or hypertonic packed cells (Dintenfass, 1964a).

2.16   EFFECT OF ANTICOAGULANT ON BLOOD VISCOSITY

The viscosity of blood remains constant at low shear rates with no anticoagulant for 2 to 4 min after removal from the circulation (Dintenfass, 1964b). Clotting starts after varying time intervals, depending not only on the intrinsic properties of the particular blood sample, but also on the shear rate used.

Blood containing citrate as an anticoagulant possesses a slightly higher apparent viscosity than blood with no anticoagulant; the use of heparin results in a slightly lower apparent viscosity.

Rosemblum (1968) divides anticoagulants into two groups:

1. Those that shrink erythrocytes – citrate and oxalate.

2. Those that have no effect on cell size or shape – heparin, ethylene diamino tetraacetic acid (EDTA), acid- citrate dextrose (ACD). Although cells shrink in citrate, they do not diminish in ACD.

Accordingly, group 1 anticoagulants increase viscosity even though citrate reduces hematocrit, while those in group 2 have no effect.

Blood in ACD can be maintained for 2 days at $4°C$ without change in viscosity, but the viscosity of blood in potassium oxalate changes in 2 or 3 hours. However, blood in "balanced" oxalate, that is, ammonium oxalate and potassium oxalate mixture (Wintrobe, 1962) and heparinized blood, is stable for 1 to 2 days at $4°C$. The amounts added are critical.

With heparin as an anticoagulant, red cells incubated at $37°C$ are crenated in 24 hours when the ATP levels are depleted. Regeneration of ATP levels by the addition of glucose, inosine, and adenine caused the cells to reassume biconcave disc shape (Hochmuth and Mohandas, 1972).

Acute heparinization has no effect on the rheological properties of dog blood (Meiselman et al., 1971). Frasher et al. (1967) prepared an external AV shunt in dogs which was used as a tube viscometer. The infusion of heparin caused no change in the apparent viscosity of blood. Neither heparin nor sodium EDTA alters blood viscosity as determined by a cone and plate viscometer (Galuzzi et al., 1964).

Wintrobe's study (1962) did not consider storage effects. Potassium oxalate in concentration of 2.5 mg/ml decreases blood viscosity, whereas heparin does not (Mayer and Kiss, 1965). It appears that conflicting results are reported in some cases. Discrepancies may be attributable to varying degrees of care given to the measuring of the anticoagulant that was added. In our laboratory the balanced oxalate (Wintrobe, 1962) has been used, successfully preventing changes up to 2 days.

2.17   EFFECT OF DEXTRAN

Although dextran is not a natural component of blood, its widespread use to influence the flow properties of blood merits some discussion. Thorsen and Hint (1950) used dextrans of various molecular weights to show that cell aggregation and sedimentation is directly related to molecular weight of colloids in the plasma. However, failure to appreciate the osmotic effects of the dextrans has narrowed the original interpretations of the *in vivo* studies in which they were employed. Low molecular weight dextran (Rheomadrodex) is said to counteract disturbances in the flow properties of blood (Gelin and Thorsen, 1961). High molecular weight dextran (greater than 80,000) increases the aggregation of red cells, and low molecular dextran causes disaggregation (Bergentz et al., 1965). Both low molecular weight dextran (m.w. 40,000 – dextran 40) and high molecular weight dextran increase the electronegativity of red cells. Low molecular weight dextran causes a decrease in cell aggregation by dilution of plasma rather than by an effect of the dextran on the cell (Groth, 1965; Wells, 1966). Cell aggregation is often measured by sedimentation or with a turbidimetric method (e.g., Engeset et al., 1967a, 1967b).

Readings from both the low shear rate Couette viscometer (GDM) and the capillary tube viscometer indicate that dextrans of molecular weight above 40,000 increase red cell aggregation and that all dextrans increase blood viscosity when compared with saline controls (Meiselman and Merrill, 1968). Furthermore, no "flow improvement" was evident with low molecular weight dextran. Infusion into humans of 10% albumin or dextran 40 decreased the hematocrit, erythrocyte aggregation (measured by sedimentation), and blood viscosity by about the same extent (Groth, 1965).

In rabbits, dextran 40 resulted in an increase in blood flow velocity that was greater than that expected from simple increase in circulatory volume, perhaps because of a decrease in blood viscosity by the hemodilution effect of the dextran. Dextran 40 has no effect *in vitro* on the aggregation of rabbit red cells, but it counteracts intravascular aggregation by increasing the speed of circulation (Engeset et al., 1967a, 1967b). When blood viscosity is increased through high molecular weight dextran (D-250), red cell velocity in the pial vessels of a mouse is not reduced, but plasma velocity is. D-250 solutions act to reduce hematocrit through their own volume and their contributions to plasma osmotic pressure. The expanded blood volume leads to an increase in blood pressure and increased shearing forces. Higher blood pressure might explain why increased blood viscosity was not accompanied by a reduction in cell velocity (Rosenblum, 1970).

Dextran 40 added to saline suspensions of erythrocytes increased the ζ potential, implying an increase in the electrostatic forces of repulsion acting between cells in such a suspension (Brooks and Seaman, 1969). Zeta potential is the charge difference between the diffuse movable charge layer surrounding a particle and the bulk of the surrounding liquid.

The ζ potential is an increasing function of dextran concentration and molecular weight (Brooks and Seaman, 1972). Above a critical concentration of dextran (or above a critical ζ potential), the erythrocytes disaggregate. The dextran concentration necessary for disaggregation is a strong function of the ionic strength of the suspending medium. This disaggregation seems to be induced by electrostatic interaction between cells (Brooks and Seaman, 1972). Increased electrostatic repulsion between cells, whatever the cause, reduces contact somewhat and results in a decrease of the low shear rate viscosity of the suspension (Eisler and Atwater, 1963).

In summary, the effect of low molecular weight dextran appears to be due primarily to plasma dilution and possibly to increasing repulsion forces between cells. In some cases dextran 40 appears to possess a specific cell-dispersing property. However, it is largely through the dilution effect that the aggregation of cells, and blood viscosity is reduced. Yet we lack an explanation of why high molecular weight dextran increases cell aggregation. Gelin et al. (1968) and Engeset et al. (1967a) disagree with Meiselman's *in vitro* study (1967) and assert that the intravascular aggregation of human and canine red cells caused by high molecular weight dextran can be reversed by low molecular weight dextran.

Hydroxyethyl starch (HES) another starch derivative used as a plasma substitute, has been compared with dextran, and it appears that low molecular weight HES is a very suitable substitute for plasma in viscosity studies; it also possess suitable colloidal activity (Cerny et al., 1968).

Viscosity of hemoglobin solution is comparable to that of serum albumin solution but lower than dextran solution with a similar molecular weight. Hemoglobin solution is a promising plasma substitute from a rheological point of view. Addition to blood at a constant hematocrit causes minimum elevation in viscosity but a significant increase in oxygen-carrying capacity. Therefore, administration may maintain oxygen capacity while diluting red cell concentration, thus facilitating blood flow and improving tissue metabolism (Usami et al., 1971). Clinical safeguards are not yet defined.

2.18   EFFECTS OF OTHER CELL COMPONENTS ON BLOOD VISCOSITY

Platelets and white cells normally have little influence on blood viscosity. Although platelet adhesion plays an important role in clotting and seems to occupy a key position in thrombus formation, platelets are present in such a small volume fraction compared with red cells that they exert little influence on blood viscosity. When red and white cells are removed, however, the strong attraction of platelets for one another can be noted (Swank, 1959).

In measuring plasma viscosity in a viscometer where an air interface exists, platelets (in contrast to red cells) markedly increase the strength of the polymolecular layer of plasma proteins (Copley and King, 1972).

Certain diseases are characterized by a large increase in white cells, which then appear to have the same effect on blood viscosity as red cells. The increase in white cells is sometimes associated with a reduced number of red cells; thus the total cell volume fraction is still in a normal range, and the apparent viscosity of blood and yield stress is normal. However, a suspension of white cells has a higher viscosity and yield stress than the same volume fraction of red cells (Steinberg and Charm, 1971).

2.19 RHEOLOGICAL PROPERTIES OF FROZEN RED CELLS

The viscosity of red cells frozen in liquid nitrogen and stored up to one year is the same as that of fresh cells (Chien et al., 1971). When tested, cells frozen in glycerol and stored for one week had the same yield stress and Casson viscosity after the glycerol had been removed and the cells had been suspended in the original plasma (Charm and Higgins, unpublished).

Example 2.1

(a) Determine the effect of a change in cell volume fraction on the viscosity of blood and on the pressure loss through a vessel 0.05 cm in diameter and 2 cm in length.

Given

temperature	$= 37^\circ C$
initial cell volume fraction	$= 0.40$
final cell volume fraction	$= 0.50$
plasma viscosity	$= 0.0140$ P
flow rate	$= 0.1$ cm^3/sec

Solution

The viscosity of blood initially is found from equation 2.8.

$$K^2 = \frac{0.0140}{1 - \alpha(0.40)}$$

where α is found from Fig. 2.9 or equation 2.5. Thus $K^2 = 0.028$ P. Using Poiseuille's equation, the pressure loss P is found from

$$0.1 = \frac{\pi}{8(0.028)2} P(0.025)^4$$

$$P = 3.67 \times 10^4 \text{ dynes/cm}^2$$

(b) At $37^\circ C$, if the cell volume fraction ϕ is changed from 0.40 to 0.50, what is the effect on blood viscosity?

Solution

From Fig. 2.9, for $\phi = 0.50$, α is 1.16. The new value for K^2 is

$$K^2 = \frac{0.0140}{1 - 1.16(0.50)} = 0.033 \text{ P}$$

This is an increase of $(.01033 - 0.028)/0.028 = 0.178$, or 17.8%. The pressure loss will increase 17.8% with this increase in cell concentration.

(*c*) Holding other factors the same, what is the effect on blood viscosity and Pressure loss in lowering temperature to 25°C?

Solution

The viscosity of blood will be increased. The value of α at 25°C is found from Fig. 2.9 to be 1.29. The change in plasma viscosity is estimated from Fig. 2.8. Assume a parallel variation in temperature for this plasma. At 37°C μ_p/μ_w (Fig. 2.8) is 1.80, whereas for this sample it is 2.0 – a difference of 0.2. At 25°C μ_p/μ_w (Fig. 2.8) is 1.65, and for the plasma under consideration here it would be 1.65 + 0.2 or 1.85. At 25°C $\mu_w = 0.009$ P and $\mu_p = 0.009 (1.88) = 0.0166$ P. The new blood viscosity is then

$$K^2 = \frac{0.0166}{1 - 1.29(0.40)} = 0.0343$$

This represents an increase of $(0.0343 - 0.028)/0.028 = 0.225$, or 22.5%.

Since the pressure drop loss in Poiseuille's equation varies directly with the increase in viscosity, the drop in temperature from 37 to 25°C causes an increase in pressure loss of 22.5% in this case.

Example 2.2

Calculate the optimum cell volume fraction for maximum cell flow rate in a tube with a constant pressure difference between entrance and end; that is, for the maximum number of cells per unit time to flow past a given point.

Solution

    Given

        Cell flow rate $\ = Q\phi$
        Total flow rate = driving force/resistance

The resistance parameter is a function of a geometry term $f(G)$, which is constant, and a viscosity term K^2, which varies with hematocrit. Combining the driving force constant and $f(G)$ into a single constant M

$$Q\phi = \frac{M}{K^2}$$

From equation 2.9 we have

$$K^2 = \frac{\mu}{1 - \alpha\phi}$$

where α is a function of hematocrit as shown by equation 2.5 or Figure 2.9. Thus we write

$$Q = \frac{M}{\mu}(1 - \alpha\phi)\phi$$

The change in cell flow rate with respect to change in cell volume is $d(Q\phi)/d\phi$. By solving for ϕ when $d(Q\phi)/d\phi = 0$, the value for ϕ making $Q\phi$ a maximum is found.

$$\frac{dQ}{d\phi} = 0 = 2\alpha\phi - \phi^2\frac{d\alpha}{d\phi}$$

Solving for ϕ using Figure 2.9 to determine α, it is found that the optimum $\phi = 0.46$, ($\alpha = 1.17$ and $d\alpha/d\phi = 0.4$).

The calculation is made by trial and error. That is, we assume a value for ϕ, taking α and $d\alpha/d\phi$ from Figure 2.9 for the assumed value of ϕ, ($d\alpha/d\phi$ is the slope of the curve), substituting values in the equation and determining whether the equation equals zero.

The value of ϕ is readjusted until the equation does equal zero. Experiments with the isolated hind paw of a dog have shown that about 46 is the optimum hematocrit at physiological pressures, but at lower pressures the optimum tends to be lower (Benis et al., 1970). This result may be due to cell aggregation occurring at the lower hematoctit. Under such conditions the relation between viscosity and cell concentration used here would be altered.

Crowell and Smith (1967), who carried out a calculation of optimum hematocrit using the data of Haynes and Burton (1959), concluded the optimum hematocrit is 40. However, a term analogous to $d\alpha/d\phi$ was omitted from their calculation, causing the discrepancy. It is interesting to note that the optimum hematocrit is a function only of the relationship between blood apparent viscosity and hematocrit.

APPENDIX   VISCOMETERS FOR BLOOD

A2.1   Cone and Plate Viscometer

The cone and plate viscometer consists of a flat plate and a rotating cone with a very obtuse angle (see Fig. 2.5a). The apex of the cone just avoids touching the plate surface, and fluid fills the narrow gap formed by the cone and plate. If the angle is small (e.g., less than $3°$), the average gap width is small, and the whole sample is subjected to constant rate of shear as in the case of the parallel plates.

Rate of shear at any point is

(A2.1) $\gamma_{(R)} = \dfrac{2\pi NR}{R \tan \psi} = \dfrac{2\pi N}{\tan \psi} \cong \dfrac{2\pi N}{\psi}$

where ψ = cone angle

N = rotational speed of cone

The shear stress is constant throughout and is

(A2.2) $\tau = \dfrac{3G}{2\pi R^3}$

where G = torque

R = radius of cone

Cone in cone viscometers have characteristics and equations similar to those obtained from cone and plate equipment.

Dintenfass et al. (1966) described a cone in cone viscometer used in studies of blood viscometry between shear rates of 0.1 to 200 $\sec^{-1}$.

The most commonly used cone and plate viscometers for blood viscometry are manufactured by the Brookfield Engineering Company. These are suitable for measurements ranging from 5 to 1500 $\sec^{-1}$.

Brookfield cone and plate viscometers are suitable for blood viscometry work, provided they are calibrated daily with a standard fluid. Reproducibility is within 2% for blood (see Section A2.8). It has been suggested that these instruments have a shortcoming in the measurement of protein solutions, since protein denatures at the air interface of the moving cone; however, such denaturation has not proved to be a major problem in measuring blood at shear rates above 1 $\sec^{-1}$. Evans et al. (1967) employed a cone and plate viscometer with a guard ring to prevent surface denaturation between shear rates of 0.1 and 125 $\sec^{-1}$. Care must be taken that settling of the suspension does not occur to a great extent during the measurement, (see A2.8).

A2.2   Coaxial Narrow Gap Viscometer

The fluid fills the narrow gap between two concentric cylinders. When the outer cylinder is turned, torque is exerted on the inner cylinder through the fluid. If the gap is sufficiently narrow (less than 5% of the radius), the velocity profile in the narrow gap is approximately a straight line. If the linear velocity of the rotating cylinder is v and gap width is δ, the velocity gradient or shear rate is v/δ. The shear stress τ exerted on the inner cylinder is

(A2.3) $\tau = \dfrac{G}{2\pi RL}$

where G = torque

R = radius of cylinder

L = length of cylinder

It is assumed that the bottom of the cylinder has no effect on the torque. To avoid end effects, the bottom of the cylinder may be indented, as in Fig. 2.5c.

Another method employed to prevent unaccountable end effects involves shaping the end of the cylinder into a cone, making the end of the cylinder a cone and plate viscometer. The cone and plate arrangement at the end of the cylinder is designed to have the same shear rate as the cylinder. The shear stress now becomes

(A2.4) $$\tau = \frac{G}{2\pi R^2 L} + \frac{3G}{2\pi R^3}$$

When measuring the viscometry of protein solutions, the air interface may cause denaturing, as has been suggested in the case of cone and plate viscometers. However, it is possible to prevent this by employing a guard ring. The guard ring is not attached to the torque system of the viscometer but yet is immersed in the fluid in a manner that prevents any fluid that reaches the air–interface from exerting influence on the torque system (see Fig. 2.6).

A2.3   Capillary Tube Viscometers

The capillary tube viscometer is most commonly used to measure blood viscometry. Although it appears to be a simple device, it is subject to a number of errors. These have been enumerated by Van Wazer et al. (1963) and are described in Table A2.1.

It is possible to express wall shear rate and stress from pressure–velocity measurements in capillary tubes by making the following assumptions (see equations 2.1 and 2.2:

1. Steady flow.
2. No radial components of velocity.
3. Axial velocity is a function of distance from axis only.
4. No slippage or marginal layer at the wall.
5. No end effects.
6. Isothermal conditions.
7. Fluid incompressible.
8. No external forces.

In applying equation 2.2 to blood viscometery, care must be taken to avoid the axial migration of cells and the subsequent formation of a marginal plasma layer (see Section 3.17). In the absence of a marginal layer, the capillary tube is a perfectly suitable instrument for blood viscometry. It is possible that

Table A2.1   Errors in Capillary Viscometry[a]

Factor	Cause	Applicability
Kinetic energy losses	Loss of effective pressure because of kinetic energy in issuing stream	General
End effects	Energy losses due to viscous or elastic behavior when a fluid converges or diverges at ends of a capillary	General
Elastic energy	Energy loss by elastic deformation of fluid not recovered during flow in capillary	Viscoelastic materials
Turbulence	Departure from laminar flow	General
Pressure losses prior to the capillary	Sticking of piston or energy dissipated in flow of material within cylinder before entering capillary	Cylinder–piston viscometers
Drainage	Liquid adhering to wall of viscometer reservoir	Glass capillary viscometers
Surface-tension effects	Variations of surface tension from one test substance to another	Glass capillary viscometers
Heat effects	Conversion of pressure energy into heat energy through flow	High-shear viscometers
Wall effects	Surface phenomena at fluid–wall interface	Polyphase fluids (some Bingham bodies and other liquids)
Effect of time-dependent properties	Variations in the residence time in capillary	Thixotropic and rheopectic materials

[a]From van Wazer et al. (1963).

60

adsorbance of proteins on the capillary wall causes a decrease in tube radius; if so, this behavior might explain the "double-layer" concept of Copley and Scott-Blair (1960).

A2.4   Kinetic Energy Correction

When a fluid discharges from a capillary viscometer directly into air, the stream carries an appreciable amount of kinetic energy. This kinetic energy may represent a significant portion of the total pressure under certain conditions. The kinetic energy loss may be calculated using the principles set forth in Section 3.14 (see equation 3.20).

By energy balance we have

$$\frac{P_1}{\rho} + \frac{V_1{}^2}{\lambda} = \frac{P_2}{\rho} + \frac{V_2{}^2}{\lambda} + \frac{\Delta P_f}{\rho} \qquad \text{or} \qquad (P_1 - P_2)\frac{1}{\rho} = (V_2{}^2 - V_1{}^2) + \frac{\Delta P_f}{\rho}$$

where ΔP_f = pressure difference due to friction
λ = 1 for streamline flow, 2 for turbulent flow
subscript 1 = entrance
subscript 2 = exit

The value of $V_2{}^2 - V_1{}^2$ determines whether the kinetic energy must be considered. When $V_2{}^2 - V_1{}^2$ is negligible compared with $(P_1 - P_2)$ $1/\rho$ the kinetic energy can be neglected.

A2.5   "End Effect" Corrections

The shape of capillary ends play an important role in determining the extent of frictional losses. Trumpet-shaped (or rounded) entrances and exits give less frictional loss than simple square ends. For blood, the entrance effect will be about 15% of the kinetic energy effect. When L/D is 150 or greater, both the kinetic energy effect and the entrance effect will be negligible compared with frictional energy loss.

A2.6   Turbulence

The equations on which viscosity is calculated from pressure–flow-rate information in capillary tubes are based on streamline flow. It is noted in Section 3.12 that when the Reynolds number for blood is greater than 800, there is deviation, due to turbulence, from streamline flow.

To calculate viscosity from pressure–flow-rate information, it is essential that the Reynolds number be less than 700.

A2.7   Surface–Tension Correction

If a capillary is narrow enough, surface tension may cause a substantial driving force to blood when air–blood interface exists in the tube.

The driving force due to surface tension σ, is $2\sigma/R_w$. A comparison of $2\sigma/R_w$ with the total pressure drop in the capillary indicate whether surface tension effects are important. An air interface with the blood in the capillary is necessary for a surface-tension effect.

In a tube with a radius of 0.01 cm, the driving force due to surface tension is about $2(70)/0.01 = 1.40 \times 10^4$ dynes/cm^2. When the capillary tube is filled with blood and there is no air–blood interface, no surface-tension effect is present.

A2.8   Operation of Wells-Brookfield Cone and Plate Viscometer: Measurement of Blood Shear Stress-Shear Rate Relationships

The viscometer is operated in air at 12 rpm. The steadiness of the indicator is observed and, if erratic, the viscometer should be checked. Also, when the viscometer is stopped, the indicator should rest at zero; if not, the viscometer should be checked again.

A standard Newtonian fluid with a viscosity of 5 to 10 C.P. is used to standardize the viscometer each day under the temperature conditions to be used. Water at controlled temperature should be circulated in the cup jacket.

The correct amount of standard fluid (it varies for each viscometer) is pipetted into the viscometer carefully avoiding bubble formation. The tip of the pipette should not touch the viscometer cup to avoid scratching the plating.

Stress readings are obtained over a range of shear rates. The ratio of the shear stress to shear rate at any speed should equal the viscosity of the standard fluid. If it does not, the screw adjustment to which the cup or plate is attached is adjusted so the ratio equals the standard fluid viscosity.

The viscometer cone and plate are gently cleaned with acetone and water to remove the oil. Care must be taken not to jar the cone which could damage the jeweled pivot.

After the cone and plate are thoroughly dried with a lint-free towel, the exact amount of blood is pipetted into the cup; it is important that no bubbles form. The viscometer is operated over the range of speeds available, first from low to high and then repeated from high to low. Readings should duplicate within one unit. The run should be completed with 5 minutes since with longer periods in the viscometer, cell-sedimentation effects influence the measurements. After the viscometer is cleaned with water, the run is repeated with a second sample of blood.

With experience and a properly operating viscometer (e.g., 0.4 RVT model) it is possible to replicate within one percent in the shear-rate range of 5 to 1500 sec^{-1}.

The viscometer is siliconized every other day when in continuous use.

After the final measurement of the day, the viscometer is again standardized to check against the earlier standardization.

Flow Behavior of Blood

Chapter 3

IN CHAPTER 2 WE DISCUSSED THE FACTORS AFFECTING blood viscosity and the measurement of blood viscosity. In this chapter the relationship between blood viscosity and flow is explained. We deal with the flow patterns influenced by blood viscosity, such as axial migration of cells and the resulting plasma layer, along with the influence on flow in branches.

Methods for calculating blood flow energy losses are presented to permit quantitative estimation of the effect of the various pertinent parameters.

3.1 LAMINAR FLOW AND FLOW EQUATION

Under most physiological conditions blood exhibits laminar flow in which streamlines of fluid slip by one another in an orderly manner (see Fig. 1.7). The complete mathematical expression describing blood in laminar flow in a straight tube is contained in the Appendix to Chapter 3. The basic differential equation is derived by considering the forces acting on a slug of fluid moving downstream in a tube.

A force due to the pressure difference along the length of the fluid acts on the cross-sectional area of the fluid mass $P\pi R^2$. An opposing and equal force acts over the lateral surface area of the slug and is $\tau 2\pi RL$ (see Fig. 3.1). Since both forces are equal, fluid moves with a constant velocity, and we have

$$(3.1) \quad P\pi R^2 = \tau 2\pi RL \quad \text{or} \quad \tau = \frac{PR}{2L}$$

Since the relationship between shear stress and shear rate of blood $- dV/dR$ is given by the Casson relationship (equation 2.8), this expression can be substituted for τ in equation 3.1. Rearranging equation 3.1 and substituting in equation 2.8, we write

$$(3.2) \quad \left(\frac{PR}{2L}\right)^{1/2} = K\left(-\frac{dV}{dR}\right)^{1/2} + C^{1/2}$$

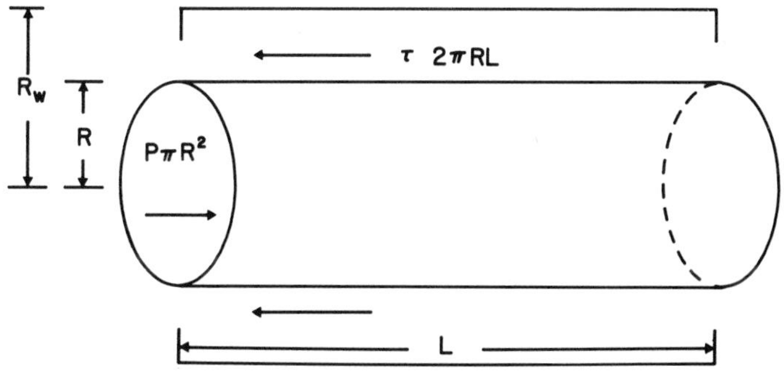

Fig. 3.1   Forces acting on section of flowing fluid.

At the wall of the tube, the velocity of flow is zero; that is, the layer of fluid next to the wall remains fixed. Even materials that do not wet the wall (e.g., mercury) have a streamline next to the wall which does not move (Hagenbach, 1860). The velocity of streamlines increases as the center of the vessel is approached from the wall.

Integration of equation 3.2 gives equation 3.3, which expresses the point velocity in the tube as a function of distance from the center.

$$(3.3) \quad v = \frac{1}{K^2} \frac{P}{4L} (R_w^2 - R^2) - \frac{4}{3K^2} \left(\frac{PC}{L}\right)^{1/2} (R_w^{3/2} - R^{3/2}) + \frac{C}{K^2} (R_w - R)$$

Equation 3.3 holds for values of R greater than $2LC/P$. When R is less than $2LC/P$, plug flow occurs; that is, the blood structure flows unsheared. The radius of the plug is

$$(3.4) \quad R_P = \frac{2LC}{P}$$

The velocity of the plug v_p may be found by substituting $2LC/P$ for R in equation 3.4. At sufficiently low pressure, the plug may clog the tube and

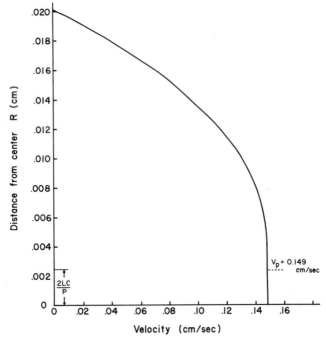

Fig. 3.2 Velocity profile for flowing blood showing effect of yield stress; see Example 3.2.

prevent flow; see Example 3.6. The flexibility of red cells and the deformability of the plug tend to prevent clogging (Tichner and Sacks, 1971). A computer program for solving equation 3.3 appears in the Appendix to Chapter 3, Fig. A3.4. An example of a velocity profile, which is a plot of equation 3.3, appears in Fig. 3.2. Proceeding to the centerline from the wall, the shear stress decreases and reaches zero at the centerline as expressed in equation 3.1. Since the size of red cell aggregates is a function of the shear stress, smaller aggregates appear nearer the wall, where the shear stress is greatest, and larger ones are observed near the centerline, where the shear stress and the shear rate are lower. The slope of the velocity profile in Fig. 3.2 is the reciprocal of the point shear rate in the vessel.

The flow rate of blood passing through the tube is determined from

$$(3.5) \quad Q = \int_{2LC/P}^{R_w} 2\pi R \, v \, dR + \pi \left(\frac{2LC}{P}\right)^2 v_p$$

where v = point velocity from equation 3.3

v_p = plug velocity found from equation 3.3 when $R = 2LC/P$

Substituting equation 3.3 for v and integrating, we see that the volumetric flow rate becomes

$$(3.6) \quad Q = \frac{\pi P}{8K^2 L}\left[R_w{}^2 - \frac{1}{2}\right)\frac{2LC}{P}\right)^2\right]^2$$

$$-\frac{8\pi}{3K^2}\left(\frac{PC}{2L}\right)^{1/2}\left\{\left[\frac{R_w^{7/2}}{2} - \frac{R_w^{3/2}}{2}\left(\frac{2LC}{P}\right)^2\right]\right.$$

$$-\frac{2}{7}\left[R_w^{7/2} - \left(\frac{2LC}{P}\right)^{7/2}\right]\right\} + \frac{2\pi C}{K^2}$$

$$\left\{\left[\frac{R_w{}^3}{2} - \frac{R_w}{2}\left(\frac{2LC}{P}\right)^2\right] - \left[\frac{R_w{}^3}{3} - \frac{1}{3}\left(\frac{2LC}{P}\right)^3\right]\right\}$$

$$+ \pi \left(\frac{2LC}{P}\right)^2 v_p$$

The mass average velocity $\overline{V}$ is related to flow rate by

$$(3.7) \quad \overline{V} = \frac{Q}{\pi R_w{}^2}$$

A computer program for solving equation 3.6 appears in the Appendix to Chapter 3 (Fig. A3.3).

When the flow rate is sufficient to cause relatively high shear stress throughout the vessel, the aggregates are small and $2LC/P$ is negligible compared with R_w. In this case, the terms in equation 3.6 containing $2LC/P$ become zero and the equation can be written in dimensionless form:

$$(3.8) \quad \frac{32K^2}{D\bar{V}\rho} = \frac{PD}{\bar{V}^2 L\rho} - \frac{16}{3}\frac{C}{\bar{V}^2\rho}\left[\frac{12}{7}\left(\frac{PD}{2LC}\right)^{1/2} - 1\right]$$

where ρ = density of blood

$D = 2R_w$

In the analysis of blood flow there are advantages in expressing equation 3.6 in dimensionless form as in equation 3.8. For example, if pressure–velocity data were plotted according to equation 3.8, all flow that is described by the model on which equation 3.8 is based would fall on a single line. Deviations from the line would indicate that this flow model did not describe the flow. The dimensionless groups help us recognize quantitatively the conditions under which deviations would be expected to occur.

When red cells are uniformly distributed throughout the tube, equation 3.6 or equation 3.8 accurately expresses blood flow. Red cells are uniformly distributed throughout when the hematocrit is 40 or greater and when the tube diameter is greater than 155 μ. Uniform distribution of cells also occurs when tube diameters are greater than 70 μ and the dimensionless group $C/\bar{V}^2\rho$ is greater than 0.01 (Charm et al., 1968a). The flow conditions in which cell distribution is not uniform are described in Sections 3.4 and 3.5.

The term $C/\bar{V}^2\,\rho$ is from equation 3.8, and its value reflects the prominence of the yield stress effect. Yield stress effects are usually negligible when $C/\bar{V}^2\,\rho$ is less than 5×10^{-4}. The smallest tube diameter to which equation 3.8 is applicable has not been determined.

When yield stress is negligible, equations 3.6 and 3.8 reduce to the dimensionless form of Poiseuille's equation (see equation 1.1). Thus Poiseuille's equation is adequate for describing blood flow when $C/\bar{V}^2\,\rho$ is less than 5×10^{-4} (C is determined by extrapolation from shear rates above 1 sec^{-1}; see Chapter 2), when tube diameter is greater than 155 μ, and when hematocrit is greater than 40.

Equation 3.6 was first proposed by Reiner and Scott-Blair (1959). A similar equation was tested by Merrill et al. (1959), who suggested that it might be employed over a wider range of conditions than Charm et al. (1968a) found to be possible.

3.2   BLOOD FLOW PATTERNS IN VIVO

A method for measuring the velocity of fast-moving cells in blood vessels was proposed by Basler (1918). A segment of the vessel is framed by a slit oriented parallel to the direction of flow, and film is run at a constant speed at right angles to the direction flow. The fast-moving cell photographs as a streak whose angle with the direction of flow is related to the cell velocity. For example, a cell moving at the same speed as the film produces a 45° angle.

Monro (1962, 1964) applied the foregoing principle in the construction of an optical system that has the advantage of permitting immediate readout of linear velocity. His modification consisted of a rotating prism set at a right angle to the direction of flow to produce the angles. The speed of the prism, which is directly proportional to cell velocity, can be measured with a tachometer.

Vessel diameter can be monitored continuously with a television scanning system for a photometric scan of the microcirculation (Wiederhielm, 1963). Diameter can also be determined continuously by use of a flying spot microscope (Johnson and Greatbatch, 1966).

Intravascular pressure can now be ascertained using pipettes 1 to 2μ in diameter and a servosystem that measures the pressure required to keep blood entering the pipette (Wiederhielm et al., 1964).

In rabbit vessels 12 to 20 μ in diameter, cells travel 0.1 to 0.5 cm/sec (Monro, 1965). The narrow column of cells is surrounded by a relatively wide zone of cell-free plasma. There is a rhythmical change in the blood velocity in an arteriole, but this has a much longer periodicity than the pulse wave – which is of the order of 10 to 30 sec, depending on the level of autonomic tone. Rabbit vessels of the 12 to 20 μ size exhibited intermittent concentration of cells followed by cell-free columns of plasma. It has been suggested that red cell velocity in the microcirculation shows pulsatile flow and can be recorded from almost all vessels larger than capillaries (Gaehtgens et al., 1970).

Intermittent corpuscular flow in rat capillaries is also noted by Palmer (1959), and a similar tendency to grouping of mammalian red cells in arterioles is visible in the high-speed photographs of Bloch (1962). Two hypotheses that have been offered to explain the intermittent nature of flow involve the rigidity of red cells and the presence of small plugs. As groups pass into finer arterioles, the red cells become deformed, and the diameter of the plastic masses may be reduced to less than the diameter of the red cell at rest.

The rigidity of the cell masses or cells influences their velocity. The more flexible cells or masses should move more rapidly (see Section 2.7). A rigid mass or cell travels more slowly, causing more flexible ones with more rapid velocity to collect behind (Whitmore, 1968). This may account in part for the intermittent concentration of cells observed. Palmer (1959) believed that leukocyte plugging in capillaries might be responsible for intermittent high and low cellular concentrations.

By the method of Monro, the mean arterial velocity in rabbit mesentery was found to be 0.6 cm/sec; in 30 to 70 μ diameter vessels, the value was 0.36 cm/sec. The mean velocity in hamster cheek pouch arterioles, averaging 34 μ diameter, was 0.44 cm/sec; in venules of 24 to 74 μ diameter, the average velocity was 0.26 mm/sec (Slechta and Fulton, 1963; Grillo and Slechta, 1963).

Another method for measuring velocity profiles in vessels of 30 to 120 μ diameter is through a modification of the photometric double-slit method for measuring erythrocyte velocities in capillaries (Wayland et al., 1967). Signals associated with the passage of red cells across the phototransistors are recorded simultaneously from double slits. Phototransistors are mounted on a screen onto which the image of the tube or vessel is projected. The small size of the phototransistors permits the investigator to arrange them to make simultaneous measurements in different positions across the same vessel, thus giving a velocity profile. Measurements made in arterioles and venules up to 70 μ diameter in the cat mesentery show midline velocities of up to 3 cm/sec in arterioles and 0.6 cm/sec in venules. Pulsatile flow is often observed in both arterioles and venules (Gaehtgens et al., 1971).

Table 3.1 presents a typical relationship between velocity and distance from the center in a 60-μ vessel of a hamster cheek pouch as measured with an instrument similar to Monro's (Berman and Fuhror, 1966).

Table 3.1   Velocity Versus Distance from Center in 60-μ Hamster Vessel[a]

R (μ)	v (cm/sec)
0.0	0.36
10	0.29
20	0.20
30−29	0.12

[a] $\phi = 0.29$, $K^2 = 0.0164$ P, $T = 37°$C, $\mu_p = 0.011$ P; the viscosity term K^2 is determined experimentally in a 500-μ tube viscometer and checked by calculation using equation 2.9.

This type of velocity profile information allows us to determine the pressure drop per unit length in the vessel and the shear rate at the vessel wall. To illustrate how this may be carried out, plot the data in Table 3.1: the slope of v versus R could be determined at some point (e.g., at $R = 20 \times 10^{-4}$ cm), and we know that the slope $-(dv)/(dR)$ is the shear rate at the given point − in this case, 90 sec^{-1}. The shear stress at that point can be estimated since, in the absence of a yield stress,

$$\frac{\tau}{-dV/dR} = K^2$$

Thus $\tau/90 = 0.0164$ P or $\tau = 1.48$ dynes/cm^2. (This stress is about 20 times greater than the yield stress for $\phi = 0.29$, and we can reasonably neglect yield stress.)

The pressure gradient can be calculated using equation 3.1; it is

$$1.48 = \frac{P}{L} \frac{20 \times 10^{-4}}{2} \quad \text{or} \quad \frac{P}{L} = 1.48 \times 10^3 \text{ dynes/cm}^3$$

The pressure gradient is the same at the wall, and the shear stress at the vessel wall is

$$\tau_w = 1.48 \times 10^3 \frac{(30 \times 10^{-4})}{2} = 2.2 \text{ dynes/cm}^2$$

Since there is probably a layer of plasma at the wall with a viscosity of about 0.011 P, the shear rate at wall γ_w is

$$\frac{\tau_w}{\mu_p} = \frac{2.2}{0.011} = 200 \text{ sec}^{-1}$$

If the fluid flowing in the vessel were Newtonian and if it followed Poiseuille's equation, the flow rate in the vessel would be 2.87×10^{-6} cm^3/sec (using the viscosity of whole blood with uniform cell distribution); from equation 3.7, the average velocity would be $\overline{V} = 0.103$ cm/sec. This value is less than any of the point velocities in Table 3.1, which is impossible. Consequently, it appears that Poiseuille's equation does not apply and a uniform distribution of cells does not exist. If plasma viscosity is used instead of blood viscosity, the average velocity is about 0.15 cm/sec.

The shear rate at the wall for a fluid in Poiseuille flow can also be found from $\gamma_w = 8\overline{V}/D$. Using 0.15 cm/sec, for $\overline{V}$, the shear rate at the wall is $8(0.15)/(60 \times 10^{-4}) = 200$ sec^{-1}. This is in close agreement with the shear rate calculated from the slope of the experimental velocity profile. The development of a marginal layer of plasma at the wall diminishes the effect of blood viscosity and would account for the increased flow rate over that predicted by Poiseuille's equation.

Estimates of wall shear rates in various vessels in man appear in Table 3.2. In large vessels, wall shear rates range between 100 and 200 sec^{-1}; in small vessels, the range is 800 to 8000 sec^{-1}. When flowing cells are frozen in place in vessels of a rabbit, it is observed that cells near the wall are preferentially oriented (Phibbs, 1967). This orientation probably influences the formation of a marginal plasma layer and might influence cells entering branches. Both a marginal plasma layer and a radial cell distribution are evident. Marginal layer widths observed by this method compare well with those calculated from Fig. 3.6 (Phibbs, personal communication 1967).

Thus several lines of evidence support the hypothesis that flow in tubes does not follow a perfect pattern of even streamlines and uniformly distributed cell concentration but rather, a layer of decreased concentration or a plasma gap exists at the wall of the vessel.

Table 3.2   Estimates of Wall Shear Rate in Various Vessels in Man
$[\gamma_w = 8(\overline{V}/D)]$

Vessel	Average Velocity[a] (cm/sec)	Diameter[b] (cm)	γ_w (sec^{-1})
Aorta	40	2.5	155
Artery	45	0.4	900
Arteriole	5	0.005	8000
Capillary	0.1	0.0008	1000
Venule	0.2	0.002	800
Vein	10	0.5	160
Vena cava	38	3.0	100

[a]Taken from Fig. 1.1.
[b]Taken from Table 1.1.

3.3   THE MARGINAL PLASMA LAYER

Poiseuille was the first to observe that a "marginal layer" was filled with plasma, and in 1835 he won a prize in experimental physiology for this work.

Many subsequent attempts have been made to quantify the effects of axial streaming or migration of cells away from the tube wall. Fahraeus and Lindquist (1929) accomplished such quantification by expressing the change in blood viscosity with tube diameter. Vejlens (1937) applied dimensional analysis to generalize the viscosity characteristics of the blood.

Bloch (1962) used photography to make direct measurement of the plasma layer in the mesenteric vessels of frogs and rats; the speed was 16 to 24 frames/sec (fps). The average gap-to-diameter ratios δ/D in frog mesentery were compared with marginal plasma layers calculated from pressure–velocity measurements in glass tubes (Charm et al., 1968a). Table 3.3 indicates agreement between the two. The frog mesentery values are the average of hundreds of measurements at such high velocities that cellular discrimination was either barely possible or not possible. The measurements in glass were also the average of many determinations, with cell volume fraction ϕ ranging from 0.30 to 0.43.

In comparing the values in the mesentery with those in glass tubes, it was assumed that the cell volume of the blood in the vessels measured by Bloch were in the same range. The δ/D measurements in rat mesenteries were similar to those found in the frog. Thus it appears that δ/D is the same for blood flowing in the mesentery of the frog and in the rat and for human blood flowing in glass tubes.

High-speed photography (480 to 7600 fps) in frog and rat mesenteries indicated an irregular marginal zone at vessel walls (Bloch, 1962), in agreement with a radial cell distribution as suggested by Bugliarello (1965) and Palmer (1965). However, not all studies have confirmed the presence of a marginal layer. For example, a quantitative study of blood flow in small tubes 130 to 800 μ in diameter indicated no evidence of a marginal layer and suggested that the cells were homogeneously distributed in flow (Merrill et al., 1965a).

The concept of the marginal plasma layer is one of the most controversial areas in blood flow. To further elucidate the question of the marginal layer, the relevant *in vitro* and *in vivo* studies are discussed in greater detail.

The marginal gap has been suggested as the cause for the decrease in apparent resistance to flow in small tubes. This decrease in blood viscosity with decreasing vessel diameter below 300 μ is called the sigma effect or the Fahraeus-Lindquist effect. Dix and Scott-Blair (1940) observed this phenomenon with clay suspensions and first referred to it as the sigma effect. Confusion has been introduced in the literature by implications that the sigma effect refers to the finite character of streamline widths due to the red cell diameter, as contrasted with the smooth velocity profile of a homogeneous fluid. The finite streamline effect may account for "sigma" phenomena in some cases (Scott-Blair, 1960), but it is only one of several possible causes. The sigma or Fahraeus-Lindquist effect is primarily due to the axial accumulation of cells, although the cell distribution is discontinuous and the cell interaction with the wall causes the hydrodynamic effect of axial accumulation (Watanabe et al., 1963).

Further evidence of axial accumulation is found in viscosity profiles plotted across small-diameter capillary tubes from observations of the cell concentrations with high-speed photography (see Fig. 3.3). As the axis of the tube is reached, the viscosity increases (Bugliarello et al., 1965). Calculated radial cell distribution and viscosity show the same characteristics (see Fig. 3.4 and Sections 3.4 and 3.5).

Using microscope photographs of stroboscopically illuminated pigmented

Table 3.3   Marginal Plasma Layers Measured in Frog Mesentery Vessels and Calculated from Flow of Human Blood in Glass Tubes

Frog Mesentery[a]		Human Blood in Glass Tubes[b]	
Diameter (μ)	δ/D	Diameter (μ)	δ/D
71−80	0.0416	71.8	0.0440
141−160	0.028	155	0.0220
241−270	0.023	256	0.0214

[a]Bloch (1962).
[b]Charm et al. (1968).

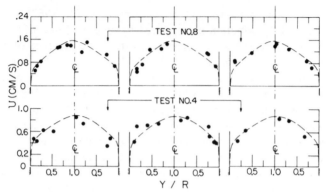

Fig. 3.3   Instantaneous velocity measurements (heavy dots) and average velocity profiles (dashed curves) in 40 m tube (from Bugliarello et al. 1965).

particles flowing in the suspension of red cell ghosts, Blackshear (1969) also found a nonuniform distribution of cells in the flowing stream. In a channel 70 μ deep, a microturbulent boundary layer thickness of about 15 μ existed at normal hematocrits.

Several experiments have been reported comparing the resistance to blood flow *in vivo* and *in vitro*. Whitaker and Winton (1934) passed blood through the hind limb of a dog and a glass tube viscometer calibrated with plasma. They concluded that there was less resistance to blood flow in the dog hind limb than in the glass and ascribed the lowered resistance to the Fahraeus-Lindquist effect.

Whitaker and Winton's experiments were repeated using freshly isolated limbs and both red cell suspensions and cell-free plasma expanders as perfusates. In addition, limbs fixed in formaldehyde were perfused with Newtonian plasma expanders of known viscosity. Essentially calibrating the system with one known Newtonian solution and measuring another Newtonian solution, large discrepancies were found among the experimental values (Benis et al., 1970).

These differences could not be accounted for on the basis of the Fahraeus-Lindquist effect. The explanation suggested by Benis et al. is that nonlinear inertial pressure losses occur in the system (e.g., exit and entrance losses associated with vessels). Generally inertial losses vary with the square of the velocity. If plasma were used to "calibrate" the *in vivo* system at a given pressure, it would flow at a more rapid rate than blood that is perfusing the system at the same pressure. Thus there would be more inertial loss associated with plasma than with blood. The flow rate of the blood in the system would then appear to be higher than expected based on the relative viscosities of blood and plasma measured outside the system. It was suggested that Whitaker and Winton neglected to consider inertial effects in their experiments (Benis et al., 1970).

However, for the inertial effects to exert such a prominent influence on the

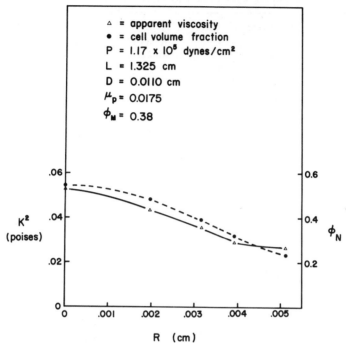

Fig. 3.4   Calculated radial distribution of cell concentration, ϕ_N (solid line) and apparent viscosity, K^2 (dotted curve).

overall pressure drop through a circulation system, they must be at least of the same order of magnitude as the viscous effects in laminar flow. (Note in Section 3.15 that entrance and exit losses do not require the viscosity term.) To have this magnitude pressure drop in a vessel 0.005 cm in diameter with a Newtonian fluid viscosity of 0.01 P and a flow rate of 5 cm/sec (average condition in an arteriole), a length of 5×10^{-4} cm would be required. However, since the average arteriole length is about 1 cm, it appears that inertial effects in arterioles are negligible.

Flowing blood in a living rat tail artery, calibrated with plasma and a radioopaque solution (200 to 500 μ) was compared with flow *in vitro*. Once more the data indicated that resistance to blood flow was less in the rat tail artery than *in vitro*. However, the decrease was more than could be accounted for by the Fahraeus-Lindquist effect (Kurland et al., 1968). Inertial effects were negligible in this case. It was suggested that differences between *in vivo* and *in vitro* cell–wall contact might explain the results.

Another possibility is the effect of electric charge on the vessel wall and the red cell. Most cells are negatively charged (Ambrose, 1965; Sawyer and Himmelfarb, 1965; Castaneda et al., 1965), and negative charged tubing affords lower flow resistance to red cells (see Table 3.4).

Table 3.4 Comparisons of Blood Viscosity Measured in Neutral Tubing and Negative Charged Tubing with Cone and Plate Viscometer

Sample	ϕ	Cone and Plate K^2 (P)	Neutral K^2 (P)	Negative K^2 (P)	Deviation (%)
M	0.44	0.0544	–	0.0439	−19.3
			0.0501	–	− 7.9
			–	0.0455	−16.4
			0.0484	–	−11.0
N	0.51	0.0552	0.0500	–	− 9.4
			–	0.0461	−16.5
			–	0.0455	−17.6
			0.0559	–	+ 1.3
			0.0603	–	+ 9.3
O	0.46	0.0544	–	0.0299	−45
			–	0.0347	−36.2
			0.0497	–	− 8.6
			0.0572	–	+ 5.2
P	0.30	0.0312	0.0273	–	−12.5
			0.0275	–	−11.9
			–	0.0298	− 4.5
			–	0.0291	− 6.7
	0.31	0.0321	–	0.0316	− 1.6
			–	0.0315	− 1.9
			0.0322	–	+ 0.3
			0.0322	–	+ 0.3
Q	0.33	0.0346	–	0.0345	0
			–	0.0315	− 9.0
			0.0346	–	0
			0.0375	–	+ 8.4
	0.37	0.0347	–	0.0352	+ 1.4
			–	0.034	− 0.9
			0.0355	–	+ 2.4
			0.0332	–	− 4.3
	0.55	0.0598	0.0580	–	− 3.0
			0.0650	–	+ 8.7
			–	0.0470	−21.4
			–	0.0464	−22.4
R	0.31	0.0347	0.0355	–	+ 2.3
			0.332	–	− 4.3
			–	0.0354	+ 2.0
			–	0.0352	+ 1.4
	0.61	0.0737	0.0699	–	−12.7
			–	0.0571	−27.5
			–	0.0569	−27.7

Since the effect of electric charge exerts an influence through relatively small distances (e.g., about 10Å), it is clear that the lower resistance in the negative charged tubing is not due simply to repulsion between cell and tube wall. It is most likely attributable to reduced contact between cell and wall or to a type of contact different from that characterizing neutral or positive charged tubes. We must also consider the type of plasma protein that is attracted to the negative charged tubing as compared with positive and neutral charge. This factor might also influence the cell—wall interaction and subsequent frictional loss. Experiments with blood flowing in negative charged polyelectrolyte capillary tubing (600-μ diameter) show about 20% lower resistance than in neutral or positive charged tubing (Ossoff and Charm, 1972); the greater the hematocrit, the greater the lowering of resistance in the negative charged tubing. With hematocrits of 30% or lower, this effect disappears in 600-μ tubing, probably because of the greater axial migration of cells and lowering of resistance in neutral tubing (see Table 3.4). Table 3.5 compares plasma viscosities measured in several types of tubing with values obtained from a cone and plate viscometer.

Reduction of surface charge of erythrocytes by neuraminidase does not alter the viscosity of these cells or their deformability as measured in a microcapillary (Seaman and Swank, 1967). This might be expected in a neutral or even a positive charged tube where the red cell charge apparently does not influence the cell—wall interaction. In a negative charged microcapillary, however, it is expected that neuraminidase would affect red cell viscosity.

Table 3.5   Plasma Viscosity Measured in Cone and Plate Viscometer Compared with Positive, Negative, Teflon, and Neutral Tubing

Sample	Cone and Plate K^2 (P)	Positive K^2 (P)	Negative K^2 (P)	Teflon K^2 (P)	Neutral K^2 (P)	Deviation (%)
S	0.0156	–	0.0147	–	–	−5.8
	–	–	–	0.0157	–	+1.0
	–	–	–	–	0.0147	−5.8
	0.0146	–	0.0135	–	–	−7.5
	–	–	–	–	0.0135	−7.5
	–	0.0147	–	–	–	+1.0

The streaming potential is the potential difference occurring when a hydrostatic pressure differential exists between the ends of a capillary, causing the flow of liquid through this capillary. The liquid phase is in motion with respect to a stationary solid phase. This condition occurs in the blood vessels of all living animals. Also of paramount importance in the quantitative study of electrokinetic effects is the concept of the interfacial or ζ potential. Zeta potential is defined as the potential at the surface of shear due to the combined effects of the charges on the surface and the equal and opposite charges of the ionic atmosphere (e.g., see Butler, 1951; Gouy, 1910).

The potential increases as the plane of shear approaches the wall surface. The streaming potential is a function of the ζ potential and is related by the Schmoluchowski equation (e.g., see Helmholtz, 1897):

$$\zeta = \frac{(4\pi\mu\kappa)}{D_e} \frac{(V_s)}{P}$$

where ζ = zeta potential

μ = viscosity (P)

D_e = dielectric constant

κ = specific conductance (stat mhos/cm; 1.07×10^{10} for blood)

P = pressure differential between measuring electrodes (dynes/cm^2)

V_s = streaming potential (mV)

Substituting various constants for blood, the equation becomes

$$\zeta = (3.02 \times 10^7) V_s/P$$

(Sawyer et al., 1965).

A few streaming potentials V_s are as follows: measured in the rabbit aorta, -12.1 mV, in the rabbit vena cava, -8.3 mV; in the rat vena cava, -10.9 mV; and in the rat aorta, -18.5 mV. The calculated potentials show that blood–internal interface is negatively charged with respect to the flowing stream (at physiologic pH), even though the Schmoluchowski equation can be applied only qualitatively to *in vivo* systems (Sawyer et al., 1965).

The *in vivo* and *ex vivo* data relative to charge on vessel walls and or streaming potential suggest that these are highly significant when flow in the microcirculation is being considered.

Bennet (1967) examined blood flow in a rectangular chamber, using a technique employing a form of Newton's interference rings by which resolution is improved at least one order of magnitude over a light microscope. He found that 60% of cells within 1.4 μ of the wall were in contact with the wall. They decrease wall contact with the subsequent formation of a thicker plasma sheath as velocity increases.

Bennet's finding brings into question classical no-slip boundary conditions, an assumed cell-free peripheral plasma sheath, or both. He suggested a more realistic model for blood flow by adding an energy-loss term based on red cell sliding contact to the usual Poiseuille flow–pressure loss. However, it has been possible to calculate pressure–flow-rate relationships for blood under appropriate conditions from experimental shear-stress–shear-rate data (Merrill, 1965), with the assumption that there is no slip at the wall. Thus it seems likely that slip action of the cells at the wall as observed by Bennet is already accounted for in the shear-stress–shear-rate data (e.g., Hyman, 1973).

Another possibility is that the slip effect exists but has a negligible effect on pressure loss. Along this line, gap widths less than 0.5 μ are calculated to have little effect on pressure–flow-rate relationships, and flow behavior is the same as if cells were in contact with the wall.

Copley (1960) observed that tubes coated with fibrin offered less resistance to blood flow than uncoated glass tubes. Plasma also exhibited less resistance to flow in fibrin-coated tubes. The same experiment was performed in Scott-Blair's laboratory and the same results were observed (personal communication with G. W. Scott-Blair, 1969). It is difficult to explain these phenomena, especially the lowering of plasma flow resistance in the context of hydrodynamic principles, since even mercury flowing in glass does not slip.

Other models describing flow in small vessels have been proposed. Poiseuille (1836) observed that the peripheral cell-free zone increased as flow rate increased. This observation on axial accumulation of red cells has been confirmed by others (e.g., Thomas, 1927 and Fahraeus, 1928). The phenomenon is not restricted to flowing red cells. A suspension of rubber discs in glycerol solution of the same density also exhibited axial migration (Muller, 1941).

The evidence for axial accumulation is both direct and indirect. Direct evidence has been obtained by microscopic visualization of "plasma skimming." Indirect evidence may be taken from the suggestion that the relative volume of cells within a tube is less than that in a bulk reservoir (Fahraeus, 1929). Similarly, the phenomenon of red cell velocity greater than that of plasma in the circulation of the living animal suggests that blood does not flow as a homogeneous suspension and that it accumulates near the axis, where velocities are greater (Dow et al., 1946; Freis et al., 1949; Rowlands et al., 1965).

The biologic usefulness of plasma skimming was proposed by Jeffery (1922), who pointed out that a suspension would flow through a tube with minimum dissipation of energy if the suspended particles were concentrated as closely as possible about the axis in the region of the minimum shear. However, Bayliss (1952) notes that Jeffery's analysis, which neglects second-order forces, does not reveal any force perpendicular to the axis of the tube; and it might well be that the force necessary to induce axial migration is due to a second-order effect.

Fahraeus (1928) showed that agglutinated red cells and the white cells of mammalian blood (which are larger than the red cells) go to the center of the tube, whereas the white blood cells of the frog (which are smaller than the corresponding red cells) remain at the edge of the axial column, suggesting that the size of flowing particles contributes to nonhomogeneity. It is now generally accepted that increased particle size favors axial drift and that the effect is most pronounced in the region near the wall.

There has been speculation on whether axial migration occurs in a uniform shear field or whether a nonuniform field is essential, the suspended particles moving out of the regions of greatest shear rate toward those of least. It was postulated that there must be a force opposing axial accumulation (Bayliss, 1952).

Taylor (1955) reported that collisions and rotation of particles in the axial stream tend to disperse the particles outward, a condition of equilibrium eventually reached when the packing tendency of the marginal zone was just balanced. The effect of such force was later quantitated by Segre and Silberberg (1962). Bayliss concluded that the formation of a marginal zone of reduced cell concentration was quantitatively inadequate to account for the reduction in the apparent viscosity of blood. This notion has since been disputed by others. In later work, Bayliss (1959, 1960, 1962) interpreted some characteristics of blood flow observed by light transmission across a tube diameter on the basis of axial accumulation of cells, although he denied its quantitative significance.

Goldsmith and Mason (1962, 1961), comparing fluid drops with rigid particles in Poiseuille flow, suggested that axial migration exists in the case of fluid drops but not with rigid particles.

Bloch noted considerable differences in the analysis of the same vessels when photographed at 480 to 7600 fps. In the control film (16 to 24 fps), the peripheral marginal layer was a sharply defined clear zone; but when the high-speed motion picture film was studied, the "layer" extended in an irregular manner toward the center of the vessel. The complex configuration changed very rapidly. Spaces or layers were interspersed by erythrocytes that slid against the wall, and a few seconds thereafter another irregular "peripheral layer" recurred. The results clearly demonstrate that the peripheral layer is in fact a statistical "cell-poor" layer.

Bloch accounted for the difference in appearance of the peripheral layer on direct microscopic examination and on high-speed film by citing the lack of contrast of the erythrocytes adjacent to wall of the vessel and a decrease in their number at the sides of the vessel, owing to volume and shallowness of the optical path. The decrease noted is coupled with the bands of plasma that extend for various distances toward the center of the vessel. The summation of these factors, according to Bloch, produces the classical peripheral plasma layer.

In further support of the idea that the plasmatic zone is an artifact is the observation by Wiederhielm and Billig (1966) — namely, that varying the angle of illumination varies the width of the marginal layer. However, this effect can be diminished if a tube of known diameter can be used as a calibrating device with the angle of illumination.

Work with tracer human red cells in transparent plasma suspensions of reconstituted biconcave ghost cells has revealed that particle crowding in tube flow results in (a) velocity distribution blunted from the parabolic and (b) particle paths exhibiting erratic radial displacements in directions normal to flow. The tube radii studied were 30 to 70 μ with velocities 0.01 to 0.6 cm/sec and 10 to 70% ghost cells (Goldsmith, 1972). The degree of blunting of the velocity profiles decreased with increasing flow rate and decreasing concentration. At low-concentration inward migration from the wall resulting in two-phase flow was significant.

In a careful photographic study of the peripheral plasma in frog mesenteries taken at 16 to 24 fps, Bloch (1962) observed that the magnitude of the plasma layer changed only with a change in flow velocity. The layer was seldom of the same magnitude on both sides of the vessel, but this discrepancy was not due to gravitational forces. As the diameter of the vessel decreased, the peripheral layer increased. In general, the peripheral layer also decreased as the linear velocity decreased.

It should be kept in mind, however, that the plasma layer is also deduced from pressure–flow-rate measurements and that the size of the deduced layer is in agreement with the direct microscopic measurements made by Bloch as noted previously (see Table 3.3). If it is assumed that this is not merely coincidence, how can it be rationalized? Perhaps the direct microscopic examination, which is relatively nondiscriminating, indicates the "time–average" configuration at the wall, whereas high-speed photography indicates the "instantaneous" configuration. Since pressure loss is a time–average result, the marginal layer deduced from pressure–flow-rate data is also a result of a time–average configuration at the wall, and this may be why it agrees in width with direct microscopic measurements at the wall.

Segre and Silberberg (1962) made the interesting observation that a rigid sphere transported in Poiseuille flow through a tube is subject to radial forces that tend to carry it to an equilibrium position at about 0.6 tube radius from the axis, irrespective of the radial position at which the sphere first enters the tubes. This is termed the "tubular pinch" effect.

Although the original observations of Segre and Silberberg were not made on blood, Taylor (1955) may have been describing the so-called tubular pinch effect when he measured the radial relative optical density in tubes with blood flowing and found a minimum transmission both near the wall and in the center.

However, Goldsmith and Mason (1962) noted that erythrocytes, because they are deformable particles, migrate toward toward the center at low flow rates (where the tubular pinch effect is negligible); moreover, the deformation effect predominates even when the flow rates are large enough to support a tubular pinch effect. Red cells form aggregates that affect results in two ways:

1. The particles are stiffer and less subject to deformation.
2. The particles are larger and more subject to axial migration.

Silberberg (1966) recorded these overlooked conditions and suggested that rouleaux could be subject to a marked tubular pinch effect in vessels 100 μ in diameter and larger.

The necessary condition for the occurrence of the tubular pinch effect is that L be greater than 0.1:

$$L = \frac{\rho \overline{V} l}{\mu} \left(\frac{a}{R_w}\right)^3$$

where ρ = density of fluid
   μ = viscosity of suspending medium
   V = mean velocity of flow
   l = length
   a = radius of particle
   R_w = radius of vessel

When $R = 300\mu$, $(a/R)_{aggregate} = 1/25$, and $L_{aggregate} = 0.09$ Thus the tubular pinch effect would move rouleaux outward, leaving the innermost core of the stream free of cells. In this sense, Silberberg remarked that the effect could be a determining factor in red cell distribution, provided the high volume fraction of the disperse phase does not introduce modification of the effects. Since the Segre-Silberberg phenomenon applies to dilute solutions, it is expected that concentrations in physiological systems would be sufficiently high to interfere with this effect.

Dilute concentrations ($\phi = 0.14$) of cells flowing in a rectangular channel 25 μ wide and 1 cm long collect berween the axis and the wall at shear rates exceeding $6000 \sec^{-1}$ (Palmer and Betts, 1972).

In some treatments, the radial force inducing red cell migration is attributed to a "Magnus effect" – a lateral deviation exhibited by spinning objects from their line of projection (Haynes, 1962; Haynes and Burton, 1959; Tollert, 1954; Saffman, 1956; Rubinow and Keller, 1961).

An example of the "Magnus effect" is the curving of a spinning baseball (see Fig. 3.5). Assume you are sitting on a spinning baseball. On one side of the ball the velocity vectors reinforce each other, and on the other side they cancel. The ball curves to the side where the velocity vectors reinforce. However, a spinning baseball in air does not represent the same pattern as a red cell flowing in a shear field where no vector cancellation occurs on one side of the cell, and the "Magnus effect" can be discounted as the reason for cell axial accumulation.

Repetti and Leonard (1966) concluded from experiments in model systems that fluid density can determine the ability of spheres to drift either way, over the entire distance from center to wall. They also observed that nonrotating spheres have the ability to drift in either direction and generally to behave like rotating particles. The effects of particle shape and deformability with respect to red cells must be considered before predictions of radial drift can be quantitative enough to be of value.

Repetti and Leonard's observation that cell rotation is not required for cell

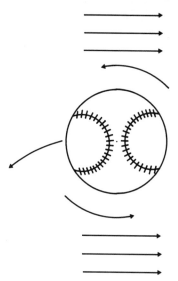

Fig. 3.5. The "Magnus effect," as illustrated by curving baseball.

drift brings to mind Vejlen's objection to the so-called Magnus effect as the cause of the inward force acting on a cell (Vejlens, 1964). In Vejlen's opinion, further evidence against the Magnus effect is provided by the conditions of blood flow in narrow vessels, where the red corpuscles are forced from the wall and transported in the axial stream at a greater distance than is supposed by the Magnus effect. There there can be no doubt that cells are caused to rotate by the stream of suspending fluid in flow and that herein lies the analogy with the Magnus effect. But this does not constitute proof that any influence of the Magnus effect is involved in the flow of the suspension.

The mutual particle interference involving red cell aggregates at the tube entrance has been suggested as a possible cause of the Fahraeus-Lindquist effect. Cokelet (1967), analyzing the data of Fahraeus and Lindquist, concluded that an entrance effect serving to reduce the mean concentration of cells in the tube could account for the change in viscosity with tube diameter. This model assumes a uniform distribution of cells in the tube, thus the absence of a marginal plasma layer. It does not explain why a high cell concentration (e.g., $\phi = 0.45$) does not result in a significant reduction of apparent viscosity in a 500-μ diameter tube, whereas a low concentration (e.g., $\phi = 0.20$) does produce a significant reduction. This can be seen in Fig. 3.6, where larger δ/D are indicative of reductions in apparent viscosity.

However, the Fahraeus effect was experimentally checked by Barbee and Cokelet in a later study (1971). The relative hematocrit inside tubes to the feed hematocrit was determined experimentally as a function of tube diameter and

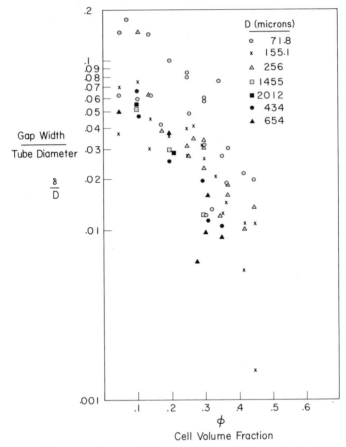

Fig. 3.6   Limiting or maximum gap/diameter ratio as a function of cell volume fraction.

feed hematocrit. Substantial changes occurred as tube diameter was reduced from 200 μ. The results of this investigation were in agreement with the Fahraeus-Lindquist effect, and the change in tube hematocrit is due to the radial distribution of cells. Fitting the Barbee-Cokelet data into the marginal plasma layer model, it is interesting to note the marginal layer width calculated from their results is in close agreement with the marginal layer widths calculated from pressure–flow rate data as indicated in Fig. 3.6. For example, in a 75-μ tube with feed hematocrit of 25%, the tube hematocrit according to Barbee and Cokelet is 19.5%. Using the equations of Thomas (1962) for calculating gap width in a plasma layer model, we find that the gap width in this case is 9.7 μ and from Fig. 3.6 for this feed hematocrit and tube diameter it is 7.5 μ. Thomas's equations are

$$\frac{H'}{H_F} = \frac{H_C}{2H_C - H_F} \qquad \text{and} \qquad \left(1 - \frac{\delta}{R_w}\right)^2 = \frac{H_F}{2H_C - H_F}$$

where H' = mean hematocrit in the tube
H_C = hematocrit of cell core
δ = marginal gap width
R_w = tube radius

The assumption in using these equations is that

$$H_C \gg H_F$$

It is proposed by Barbee and Cokelet, 1971b, that the Fahraeus effect is identified when it is erroneously assumed that the hematocrit of blood flowing in small-diameter tubes is equal to the feed hematocrit or when the radial distribution of cells is neglected. If the tube hematocrit rather than the feed hematocrit is employed, it is possible to predict the flow behavior in small tubes from the flow behavior in a large-diameter tube. However, hematocrit is an expression of a static condition, not of flow. The flow information reflected in the tube hematocrit depends on the flow model assumed.

Vand (1948) hypothesized that since a particle center cannot approach the tube wall to a distance less than half the effective diameter of the particles, a reduced concentration near the wall must result. This is known as the mechanical exclusion effect or Vand effect.

A. D. Maude and R. L. Whitmore (1958, 1956) have demonstrated that Vand's theory accounts adequately for changes in the viscosity and concentrations observed in particulate suspensions flowing through narrow tubes.

Navari and Gainer (1968) tested the effect of the marginal gap width on apparent viscosity of blood using Vand's equation (Vand, 1948) and the gap width determined from Haynes's data (Haynes, 1962). Vand's equation is

$$\frac{\mu_p}{\mu_s} - 1 = \left(1 - \frac{2\delta}{D}\right)\left(\frac{\mu_p}{\mu_x} - 1\right)$$

where μ_s = true or reservoir viscosity of suspension = K^2
μ_p = suspending fluid viscosity
μ_x = observed viscosity in capillary tube

Excellent agreement was recorded for hematocrits between 30 and 60, and the reduction in apparent viscosity was observed and calculated as tube diameters were reduced to 200 μ. Navari and Gainer did not test the hypothesis in smaller tube diameters.

Seshadri and Sutera (1968) studied the flow of neutrally buoyant spheres in water−glycol solutions and calculated the average concentration of spheres in a tube. They used an equation developed by Thomas (1962) (see equation 3.24) and assumed a gap width associated with the "wall exclusion effect," described by Maude and Whitmore (1956), of $D_p/4$, where D_p is particle diameter. They found that the flowing particles are so distributed that they travel faster in a tube than the fluid associated with them while they are in the reservoir; thus the average concentration in the tube is less than in the reservoir. Rowlands et al. (1956) noted the same distribution in a living system.

Seshadri and Sutera found that the wall exclusion effect can account for more than 50% of the particle average concentration reduction. The larger the spheres, the better the agreement with equation 3.24. They also noted that the concentration reduction (or the gap width) increased with flow rate at low flow rates and eventually approached a limiting value at higher flow rates. This change with flow rate is in agreement with quantitative measurements of gap width for blood flow in capillary tubes (Charm et al., 1968a). Although shape of the vessel had no effect on concentration reduction, Seshadri and Sutera point out that this does not prove that the entrance geometry has no effect on the radial distribution of particles in the tube.

With no hypothesis other than those usually employed in hydrodynamics, Nubar (1966) has shown that the change from a straight-line velocity profile at the entrance to a quasi-parabolic profile in developed flow downstream could cause "axial drift" of cells. Maintaining flow continuity for a streamline shell of cells, as its velocity increases with flow development, requires that the radius of the shell decrease; thus "axial drift."

Employing dilute solutions of red cells, Goldsmith (1967) examined the theory that when additional disturbances in the flow around a deformable particle are reflected off the wall, they may give rise to an inwardly directed force. He compared the velocity profiles and radial concentrations of normal cells with hardened cells and observed less inward migration with hardened cells (Goldsmith, 1968). The normal cells suspended in saline solution were examined in a 75-μ diameter tube with a wall shear rate in the order of 3300 sec^{-1} or a velocity of 0.32 cm/sec, since the wall shear rate can be approximated by $8\bar{V}//D$. The cell concentration was about $\phi = 0.01$ and the clear marginal layer that developed 4.8 cm from the tube entrance was about 15 μ. The gap to diameter ratio was $\delta/D = 0.2$. – essentially the gap width that would be found from Fig. 3.6, which was calculated from pressure–flow-rate determinations (Charm et al., 1968a).

At particle Reynolds numbers too low to cause radial migration of hardened red cells, normal red cells close to the wall migrate inward. As the Reynolds number increases, both hardened and normal cells exhibit the two-way lateral migration of the tubular pinch effect (Section 3.2), although the equilibrium radial position of the deformable cells is closer to the tube axis than for the hardened cells (Goldsmith and Mason, 1971). Goldsmith (1967) also studied the motion of rouleaux in a parabolic velocity field and explained the bending and rotation characteristics in terms of the stresses acting on the rouleaux and their mechanical properties.

In summary, the forces causing axial migration of cells in flow are not well defined. The shape, size, deformability, concentration, and flow rate of cells influence the degree of axial migration. In the microcirculation, cells do not necessarily move in a straight path but frequently bounce from the wall, suggesting that the so-called plasma layer is in fact statistical.

3.4   DISTRIBUTION OF RED CELLS ALONG THE RADIUS

In Section 3.3 it was concluded that blood sometimes flows with a nonuniform cell distribution across a tube or vessel radius. One of the major efforts at quantitating this effect was carried out by measuring the hematocrit drawn from side branches of a rectangular channel 35 μ wide (Palmer, 1965). It was also deduced that the hematocrit distribution varied linearly across the tube. The equation expressing the distribution of cell concentration when adapted to cylindrical tube is

$$(3.9) \quad \phi_R = \phi_M + A \left(\frac{2Q_{R_w \to R}}{Q_T} - 1 \right)$$

where $Q_{R_w \to R}$ = volume flow rate between wall and distance R measured from center

Q_T = total flow

ϕ_M = cell volume fraction in reservoir

A = function of cell volume fraction ϕ_M in reservoir (see Fig. 3.7)

ϕ_R = cell volume fraction associated with streamline at R

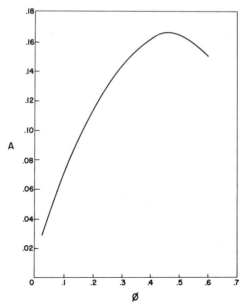

Fig. 3.7. A as a function of ϕ for calculating radial cell distribution (adapted from Palmer, 1965).

The cell distribution suggested by Palmer can be used to calculate the flow-rate–pressure relationships for blood flow when neither equation 3.6 nor 3.8 nor simple laminar flow with yield stress effects applies, but axial migration does occur. The results are in close agreement for a wide range of conditions (see Example 3.1). When hematocrit is less than 40 and $C/V^2\rho$ is less than 5×10^{-4}, the radial cell distribution is stable with respect to velocity.

Under this hypothesis, the flow rate is found by considering the volume flow rate associated with each streamline in the tube and assuming that it has a finite thickness ΔR, approximately 4 μ. The thickness ΔR is selected such that when it is divided into R_w, $R_w/\Delta R$ is a whole number. (The thickness of a laminae ΔR is not critical as long as it is taken small enough.) The laminae appear as telescoping incremental cylinders. The flow rate of each lamina or incremental cylinder is summed to obtain the total flow rate. This total flow rate or the associated pressure drop is compared with a known flow rate or pressure drop in a trial and error solution (see A3.1, and Example 3.1A).

3.5 CALCULATIONS USING MARGINAL LAYER OF PLASMA MODEL

Calculation of blood flow when cell concentrations vary along the radius is complex. It is convenient to assume the model of a cell-free marginal plasma layer at the wall, surrounding a core of cells as described previously, somewhat simplifying the more accurate model of cell distribution along the radius. This approximation does not introduce any serious error in calculating blood flow rates and pressure losses in glass capillary tubes (Charm et al., 1968a).

If the stress along the radius does not exceed the yield stress, an unsheared plug of cells exists in the central regions. These would be surrounded by a sheared plug of cells, which is in turn surrounded by an annulus of plasma. Quantitatively, the relation is conveniently expressed by

$$(3.10) \quad \frac{32K_1{}^2}{D\overline{V}\rho} = \frac{PD}{V^2\rho L} \left[\frac{[1 - (1 - 2\delta/D)^4]}{1 - \alpha\phi_1} + \left(1 - \frac{2\delta}{D}\right)^4 \right]$$

$$+ \frac{C}{V^2\rho} \left(1 - \frac{2\delta}{D}\right)^3 \left[\frac{16}{3} - \frac{64}{7} \left(\frac{PD}{2C_1L}\right)^{1/2} \left(1 - \frac{2\delta}{D}\right)^{1/2} \right]$$

where $K_1{}^2$ is the square of Casson viscosity or the limiting apparent viscosity of core of cells or

$$Q = \frac{\pi P R_w{}^4}{8L\mu_p} \left[\left(1 - \left(1 - \frac{\delta}{R_w}\right)^4\right) + \left(1 - \frac{\delta}{R_w}\right)^4 (1 - \alpha\phi_1) \right]$$

$$+ \frac{C_1\pi R_w{}^3(1 - \alpha\phi_1)}{16\mu_p} \left[1 - \frac{\delta}{R_w}\right]^3 \left[\frac{16}{3} - \frac{64}{7} \left(\frac{PR_w}{C_1L}\right)^{1/2} \left(1 - \frac{\delta}{R_w}\right)^{1/2} \right]$$

The concentration of cells in the core is

(3.11) $\quad Q\phi = Q_1\phi_1$

where Q_1 = flow rate of core
$\quad\phi_1$ = cell volume fraction of core
$\quad Q$ = flow rate in reservoir
$\quad\phi$ = cell volume fraction in reservoir

We also have

(3.12) $\quad Q_1 = Q - Q_g$

where Q_g is the plasma flow rate in the gap.

In addition, considering the velocity profile in the marginal gap, it can be shown that

$$(3.13) \quad Q_g = \frac{\pi P}{2\mu_\rho L}\left[\frac{R_w^2}{2} - \frac{(R_w - \delta)^2}{2}\right]^2$$

Modifying the equation developed by Thomas (1962), the volume fraction of cells *in* the moving core (but not the volume fraction leaving the tube) is

$$(3.14) \quad \frac{\phi_1}{\phi} = \frac{1 + [1 - (1 - 2\delta/D)^2]^2}{(1 - 2\delta/D)^2 \, 2[1 - (1 - 2\delta/D)^2] + (1 - 2\delta/D)^2 \, (1 - \alpha\phi_1)}$$

where α is found from equation 2.5.

The value of δ/D is obtained as a function ϕ from Fig. 3.6 when $C/\overline{V}^2\rho$ is less than 5×10^{-4}; that is, the marginal is fully developed.

When $C/\overline{V}^2\rho$ is between 10^{-2} and 5×10^{-4}, δ/D is obtained from

$$(3.15) \quad \log\frac{C}{\overline{V}^2\rho} = \frac{(\delta/D)_v}{(\delta/D)_m}\,[\log 5 \times 10^{-2}] + \log 10^{-2}$$

where $(\delta/D)_v$ = gap/diameter ratio when it is a function of velocity
$\quad(\delta/D)_m$ = maximum value of gap/diameter ratio occurring when $C/\overline{V}^2\rho$ is less than 5×10^{-4}.

When $C/\overline{V}^2\rho$ is greater than 10^{-2}, the marginal layer disappears and (δ/D) or δ/R_w is zero in equation 3.10 (see Example 3.2).

Under these conditions equation 3.10 may be reduced to approximate equation 3.8. It is only approximate because equation 3.10 has second-order terms that are dropped for simplification. The complete equation appears in the Appendix to Chapter 3.

A computer program for solving equation 3.10, when the gap width δ is fully developed, appears in the Appendix to Chapter 3, Fig. A3.2.

When both yield stress C and marginal layer δ are negligible, equation 3.10

reduces to the equivalent of Poiseuille's equation. An illustrative calculation using this model appears in Example 3.1b.

In the Fahraeus-Lindquist experiments (see Fig. 1.8), where a decrease in apparent blood viscosity occurs with decreasing tube diameter below 300 μ, the wall shear stress ranged between 80 and 130 dynes/cm^2 and wall shear rates from 2600 to 4300 sec^{-1}. The decrease in viscosity associated with decreasing tube diameter is thought to be due to the development of a marginal layer.

The equation expressing the point velocity or velocity profile for the marginal plasma layer model for blood flow is

(3.16)   IN THE CORE OF CELLS

$$
v_1 = \frac{P}{4\mu_p L} \left[R_w^2 - (R_w - \delta)^2\right] + \frac{1}{K_1^2} \left\{ \frac{P}{4L} \left[(R_w - \delta)^2 - R^2\right] \right.
$$

$$
\left. - \frac{4}{3} \left(\frac{PC}{L}\right)^{1/2} \left[(R_w - \delta)^{3/2}\right] + C[(R_w - \delta) - R]\right\}
$$

where R varies from $(R_w - \delta)$ to zero at the center.

(3.17)   IN THE PLASMA LAYER

$$
v_p = \frac{P}{4\mu_p L} \left[R_w^2 - R^2\right]
$$

where R varies from R_w at the wall to $(R_w - \delta)$; see Figs. 3.8a and 3.8b and the computer program for equation 3.16 in the Appendix to Chapter 3, Fig. A3.5.

Table 3.6 indicates the appropriate equations for calculating blood flow-rate—pressure relationship under various conditions.

Table 3.6   Summary of Equations for Calculating Flow Rate or Pressure Loss Under Various Conditions

Diameter (μ)	ϕ	$C/\overline{V}^2 \rho$	Equations for Calculating Flow Rate or Pressure Loss
50–2000	<0.40	<5 x 10^{-4}	3.10
50–2000	<0.4	10^{-2} to 5 x 10^{-4}	3.10 with 3.15
50–2000	<0.4	>10^{-2}	3.8 or 3.6
50– 155	>0.4	<5 x 10^{-4}	3.10
50– 155	>0.4	10^{-2} to 5 x 10^{-4}	3.10 with 3.15
50– 155	>0.4	>10^{-2}	3.8 or 3.6
155–2000	>0.4	<5 x 10^{-4}	3.8 or 3.6 or Poiseuille's equation – 1.1
155–2000	>0.40	>5 x 10^{-4}	3.8 or 3.6

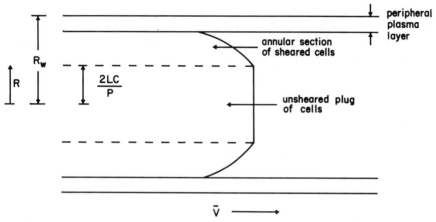

$\bar{V}$ ⟶

Fig. 3.8a   Velocity profile with marginal layer and yield stress effect; see equations 3.16 and 3.17.

The quantitation of blood flow described here recognizes three flow regions based on values of the dimensionless group $C/\bar{V}^2 \rho$, namely:

1. Low flow when $C/V^2 \rho$ is greater than 0.01 and the cells are uniformly distributed throughout the tube.

2. Intermediate flow when a marginal plasma layer or a cell-poor region at the vessel wall exists and increases with increasing flow rate when $C/\bar{V}^2 \rho$ is between 10^{-2} and 5×10^{-4}.

3. High flow rate when the marginal plasma layer has reached its maximum width with $C/\bar{V}^2 \rho$ less than 5×10^{-4}.

These flow regimes may perhaps be defined by other dimensionless groups (e.g., Reynolds number).

Merrill et al. (1965a), observing flow through a microscope, described the following four flow regimes:

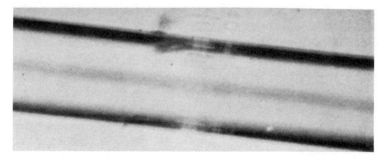

Fig. 3.8b   Flow of 1% red cell suspension in 70-μ tube. Flow rate 3×10^{-6} cm^3/sec (100X). From Charm et al. (1968).

1. At shear rates between approximately 160 and 1600 sec^{-1}, the speed of flow precludes observation of individual cells. As flow slows to values of the order of approximately 40 to 80 sec^{-1}, the cellular nature of cells becomes visible, and individual cells can be seen rolling along the walls of the tube. In this regime the cells flow as individuals without aggregates.

2. As the flow decreases to a shear rate about 8 sec^{-1}, a transition occurs to a different type of flow mechanism. The cells gather into large clumps as the flow slows even more. The flow is no longer one of individual cells, but of large tumbling aggregates.

3. As the flow rate keeps on decreasing, the red cells continually form larger and larger aggregates. Finally, the aggregates form a single network of cells and the cells travel through the tube slowly as a single plug. This appears to occur at shear rates of 0.08 sec^{-1}.

4. It is further noted that since blood exhibits a yield shear stress, theory predicts a complete cessation of flow at pressure drops at which the wall shear stress is equal to the yield stress. This point was experimentally determined by pressure–decay measurements (i.e., after flow ceases, the finite residual pressure in the tube is measured). With this procedure, cells must be in contact with the wall. However, it has been noted that the adherence of cells to walls of tubes is inconsistent. A number of investigators have observed that at very low flow rates a clear zone of plasma can be seen at the vessel wall, but this zone disappears as the cells disperse with increasing flow rate.

3.6   TAPERED VESSELS

Many blood vessels have the characteristics of tapered cylinders rather than straight cylinders. Conveniently for the purpose of calculating energy loss, we can think of the tapered cylinders as being composed of elements of straight cylinders (Charm and Kurland, 1967); see Fig. 3.9). The equation used by Cerny and Walewander (1966) to describe blood flow in a tapered vessel is reducible to

$$(3.18) \qquad \frac{\pi}{8\mu Q}(P_2 - P_1) = \int_{L_1}^{L_2} \frac{dL}{R^4}$$

In the case of a nonuniform taper $\int dL/R^4$ can be determined graphically. Cell distribution appears to develop in tapered tube segments in the same manner as in straight tubes of the same diameter. In small-diameter (300 to 70 μ) tapered glass capillary tubes, experimental values were within 5% of calculated values when marginal plasma layers were considered; when such layers were neglected, differences between calculated and experimental results were 35% (see Table 3.7, Charm and Kurland, 1967).

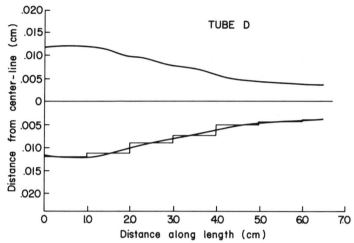

Fig. 3.9   Nonuniform tapered tube made up of segments of uniform straight tubes.

Equation 3.18 applies only to Newtonian fluids in Poiseuille flow. For blood, the pressure drop in each element must be treated as a separate problem based on the conditions in that element (see Example 3.5).

In bell-shaped constrictions (25% original area), eddy currents develop downstream when the Reynolds number is greater than 9.9. Eddy currents develop in enlarged sections when the Reynolds number is greater than 25. Eddies reduce flow rate for a given pressure and may create a potentially disastrous situation in terms of blood coagulation or platelet disposition (Lee and Fung, 1971).

Benis and Lacoste (1968b) have noted the effect of vessel taper on flow reversal in the microcirculation. Flow reversal may occur in two vessels

Table 3.7   Flow in Tapered Tube:[a] Experimental Pressure Losses Versus Calculated Losses with and without Consideration of Marginal Layer

Flow Rate (cm^3/sec)	Experimental (dynes/cm^2)	ΔP Calculated with Gap (dynes/cm^2)	Difference (%)	ΔP Calculated without Gap (dynes/cm^2)	Difference (%)
15.58×10^{-4}	541,000	566,570	4.6	707,184	31.0
9.64×10^{-4}	330,000	352,490	6.6	447,840	35.5
6.57×10^{-4}	225,000	240,000	6.6	310,374	38.0
3.175×10^{-4}	120,000	116,900	2.5	157,924	31.6

[a]Tube number D, $\phi = 0.20$, temperature = 24°C, largest diameter = 260 μ, smallest diameter = 78 μ.

connected by a shunt when the flow rate is such that the yield stress effects in one vessel exert a prominent effect on pressure drop in that vessel but not in the other one. This is most likely to occur in tapered vessels. For example, when a critical flow rate is reached such that the shear stress at some point in a tapered branch equals the yield stress (i.e., $PD/4L = C$), flow through that branch ceases; see Example 3.6. When this occurs, flow is diverted through the second branch or shunt.

For the flow of blood through a uniform tapered tube, Benis and Lacoste suggested the equation

$$(3.19) \quad \frac{PD_{LM}}{4L} = C + \frac{D_{LM}}{D_{NM}{}^4} \frac{64K(2QC/\pi)^{1/2}}{D_1^{-3/2} + D_2^{-3/2}} + \frac{D_{LM}(128)K^2Q}{\pi D_{NM}{}^4}$$

where $D_{LM} = (D_2 - D_1)/\ln(D_2/D_1)$
$D_{NM}{}^4 = 3(D_2 - D_1)/(D_1^{-3} - D_2^{-3})$.

Equation 3.19 is appropriate when marginal plasma layers do not exist in a uniform tapered tube.

3.7   FLOW IN BRANCHES

Red cell flow to a branching vessel is somewhat more complex than the same phenomenon in a straight section. The flow entering a branch from a lead vessel is greatly influenced by the cell distribution across the radius in the lead or main vessel. The pressure difference between the entrance and exit of the branch is the driving force for flow in the branch. Pressure at the branch entrance is determined by the flow conditions in the main vessel. The flow pattern and radial cell distribution governs the hematocrit or cell volume fraction entering the branch and in this way regulates the blood viscosity in the branch.

In considering branch flow, the marginal layer model is less satisfactory for analysis of the main vessel flow than the radial cell distribution model.

The flow entering the branch is not drawn symmetrically from the lead vessel but from the regions nearest the branch entrance. Illustrating this is Fig. 3.10, which presents a cross section and longitudinal view of streamlines entering a branch. A chord AB drawn in the cross section of the main vessel defines the boundary for the streamlines that will enter the branch and those that will continue downstream in the main vessel (see Fig. 3.11). Now it is clear that since each streamline in the lead vessel has a different cell concentration and velocity, these elements must be integrated in the segment defined by the chord to find the flow rate and hematocrit entering the branch.

In Section 3.5 it was noted that when $C/\overline{V}^2\rho$ was less than 5×10^{-4}, the radial cell distribution was fully developed, whereas when it was greater than 10^{-2},

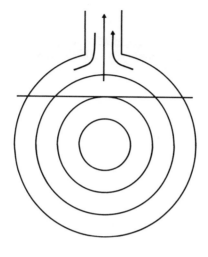

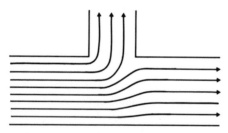

Fig. 3.10   Streamlines flowing from lead
vessel to branch (front and side views).

there was no radial cell distribution and the cell concentration was uniform
throughout the vessel. Although this concept has not been thoroughly tested, it
has been found to apply in a number of *in·vitro* experiments (Charm et al.,
1968a). Certainly in the regions where flow has almost stopped, marginal plasma
layers have also been observed. However, since there is no other quantitative
information available, this empirical observation is employed in the analysis of
branching flow.

It has also been suggested that when $C/\overline{V}^2 \rho$ is less than 5×10^{-4}, yield stress
effects are negligible and the viscosity of blood is simply its limiting apparent
viscosity of K^2.

In the radial cell distribution model, streamlines were assumed to have a finite
thickness ΔR (see Section 3.4). The calculation of the flow rate and cell volume

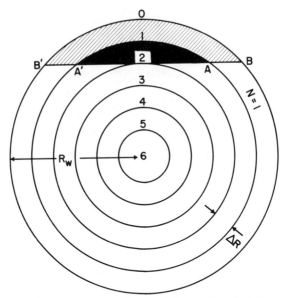

Fig. 3.11. Cross section of finite streamlines and diagram for calculating volume fraction associated with branching flow. The shaded area defined by chord $B'B$ indicates cross section entering the branch; see Sections 3.7, 3.8 and 3.9.

fraction associated with each streamline in the main vessel was described in Appendix A3.1 and Example 3.1.

Fractions of certain streamlines from the main vessel enter the branch. By determining that part of each streamline entering the branch, the flow rate and cell volume fraction in the branch are calculated.

3.8   MAIN VESSEL FLOW THAT ENTERS BRANCH

It was previously noted that the flow entering a branch is confined to a segment defined by a chord in the main vessel (see Fig. 3.11). The fraction of each streamline contained within the segment must be determined, and in finding the flow that will enter the branch, the flow rate associated with that part of each streamline is assumed. Knowing the pressure drop along the branch, the correct flow rate is calculated (see Appendix to Chapter 3 and Example 3.7).

In the living circulation, the configuration at the branch entrance influences the cell distribution and the flow entering the branch. For example, projections or "cushions" at the branch entrance may force cells toward the centerline, reducing the number admitted to the branches. In addition, the branch angle with the main vessel affects flow entering the branch through the energy or pressure loss associated with passage through the entrance.

3.9   CALCULATION OF FLOW RATE ASSOCIATED WITH A SEGMENT OF THE CROSS SECTION OF LEAD VESSEL

If the flow entering the branch is considered in cross section, it appears to be taken from a circular segment of the main vessel (see Fig. 3.10). Portions of several streamlines contribute to the flow rate associated with the segment.

Each streamline appears as an annulus when the main vessel is viewed in cross section. A part of an annulus represents that portion of streamline that enters a branch, the remaining portion of the annulus contributing to the flow in the main vessel downstream from the branch. The total flow entering the branch appears in the main vessel as a circular segment made up of parts of annuli representing several streamlines.

The calculation of areas associated with portions of streamline annuli and segments making up the flow entering the branch is described in the Appendix, A3.1.

3.10   CALCULATION OF FLOW RATE IN THE BRANCH

In the first approach to calculating flow rate in a branch it is assumed that disturbances at the branch entrance do not seriously disrupt the flow pattern in the lead vessel. The driving force for flow entering the branch is determined by the pressure difference at the entrance to the branch and the exit from the branch. The same pressure drop must exist along the main vessel after the branch. The flow divides, and thus the two pressure drops are the same. This principle is used in calculating the branch flow; see Example 3.7.

The branch angle with the lead vessel may affect the pressure drop across the entrance to the branch. A more important effect on branch flow involves the diameter of the entrance and the effect of projections in the mainstream that disturb cell distributions and flow patterns. The analysis of branch flow in the Appendix A3.1 assumes no disturbance of the flow pattern at the branch junction.

Krovetz (1963) investigated the effect of vessel branching on hydrodynamic stability, using glass models of single branches 0.3 cm in diameter whose angle varied from 15 to 150°. By observing dye, he was able to determine that laminar flow in the prebranch vessel became turbulent after passing the junction. First, shortly after reaching the branch, the dye front became tortuous and irregular; finally, as it moved down the main arm, the front was turbulent. The dye entered the branch itself only after a considerable delay, which is clearly related to the axial centering of the dye stream during laminar flow; in addition, only the fluid available along the edge near the branch contains no dye. (This dye-free area appears to be analogous to the plasma-skimming or the marginal plasma layer at the wall in suspension flow.) The phenomenon is observed even though the flow is unstable after passing the junction.

When the flow is turbulent in the prebranch (i.e., when the streamlines are disordered in contrast to the orderly pattern of streamline flow), the dye enters the branch in the same concentration as in the prebranch. The angle of branch had little effect.

Krovetz also checked the effects of branching under more physiological conditions. Dye was injected into a catheter lying in the superior vena cava, right atrium, left ventricle, aortic root, or descending aorta of a dog. Blood was withdrawn from both iliac arteries, and concentrations were noted. No differences were observed between the iliac arteries. Thus the dye is adequately mixed, as evidenced by the comparabilities of cardiac outputs from the iliac arteries. Helps and McDonald (1954) studied flow patterns in veins and found similar stability at the junction of two iliac arteries.

It has also been found that flow of neutrally buoyant spheres in branch systems (D = 6.32 mm, particle diameter = 600 μ) shows no difference between 45 and 90° branch angles (Bugliarello and Hsiao, 1964). However, when the side branch is narrower (e.g., half main branch), it appears that contributions to the branch flow come from farther across the main branch. The same investigators observed a low particle concentration in the branch with low flow rates. The concentration in the branch increased as branch flow rate increased. The change in branch concentration with flow rate is compatible with the distribution of cells across the radius, since the flow in the branch is usually drawn from the "particle-poor" layers next to the wall.

One of the best series of branch flow experiments for blood in small branch systems was carried out by Gelin (1963). These experiments were concerned with the influence of changes in the physical state of blood on the flow pattern of blood in branching capillary tubes. The apparatus consisted of two pieces of 5-mm thick Plexiglas made in exactly the same dimensions. Semicylindrical channels were made in the two pieces using an engraving technique – one longitudinal or central piece and another at a 90° angle such that the distances from the cross of the channels was exactly the same. When the two pieces were fitted together and compressed by a screw device, the semicylindrical channels formed cylinders. The channels were manufactured with diameters ranging from 500 to 110 μ. It was possible to measure the hematocrit in the branches under a variety of conditions. Plasma skimming was observed in branches and in the inlet capillary when cells aggregated. In the outlet capillary, a slow flow without plasmal skimming was observed. Possibly the flow in the outlet capillary was sufficiently slow to prevent the formation of a marginal layer (see Section 3.4).

Unfortunately Gelin did not measure blood viscosity. By estimating this value, however, it is possible to compare his experimental results with calculations. Close agreement is found; see Example 3.7. From microscope examinations, Gelin observed disturbances of the flow pattern at branch junctions.

McDonald and Potter (1963) noted laminar flow in the basilar artery of the rabbit, which is only 0.6 mm in diameter. Dye streamlines from one vertebral artery were seen to hug the ipselateral wall of the basilar artery, and no disturbances were recorded at the junction.

The calculation of branch flow as illustrated in Example 3.7 does not consider the effect of disturbance of the flow pattern at the branch junction. If this disturbance is severe enough to affect the cell concentration radial distribution, the model will be inaccurate for branch flow calculations. However, the calculations could serve as a reference frame for studying quantitatively the nature of the disturbance at the junction.

3.11 PULSING FLOW IN THE MICROCIRCULATION

McComis et al. (1966) noted that blood pulsing in flow in tubes 70 to 300 μ in diameter had the same energy loss for the time—average flow rate as would have been calculated from steady flow equations. The pulse studied was a sine wave with frequency varying from 1800 to 7200 Hz. Marginal layers appeared to develop as in steady flow.

It is confirmed from pulsatile flow studies in tubes down to 40 μ in diameter that:

1. Peripheral plasma layer dimensions are the same for steady and pulsatile flow.

2. Pulsatile velocity profiles are in phase with the pulsatile pressure gradient.

3. The average pressure drop for a given flow rate is the same for pulsatile and steady flow (Bugliarello and Sevilla, 1970).

Pulsing flow as it exists in the large vessels is usually damped out by the time it reaches the smaller vessels in the microcirculation (Burton, 1965). In spite of the great damping of the pulse wave in the arterioles, pulsation in the capillary bed can be observed; it is usually slight, however.

Blood possesses viscoelastic properties in the time scale of normal pulse rates (Thurston, 1972). These properties are dependent on the frequency and amplitude of shear rate in oscillatory flow. Stress is resolved into a viscous component τ', which is in phase with the shear rate or velocity gradient γ and an elastic component τ'', which is 90° out of phase. Plasma does not possess an elastic component. At small velocity gradients both τ' and τ'' are directly proportional to γ. For blood at $\phi = 0.50$, this character changes near $\gamma = 1 \sec^{-1}$, at a frequency of 1 Hz. At high gradients (i.e., $\gamma > 60 \sec^{-1}$), τ' again approximates a linear dependence on γ, and τ'' becomes insensitive to γ. At low γ, where linear conditions exist, the term τ'/γ shows a general decrease with increasing frequency in the range of 0.1 to 100 Hz, thus denoting a wide spectrum of relaxation times.

Pulsed flow in small capillary tubes (e.g., McComis et al., 1967; Bugliarello, 1971) did not exhibit the viscoelastic effect observed by Thurston, possibly because of the relatively high shear rate associated with this tube flow.

3.12   TURBULENT FLOW

Blood flow is usually considered to be streamlined in the microcirculatory system. Under certain conditions, however, flow changes from streamline or laminar to turbulent. In turbulent flow the streamlines turn into one another in a disorderly manner, as contrasted with the order of streamline flow (see Fig. 1.3).

The criterion for determining whether turbulent flow or streamline flow exists in the case of homogeneous Newtonian fluids is the evaluation of a dimensionless number known as the Reynolds number (Re). The Reynolds number is $D\bar{V}\rho/\mu$ where D is diameter, $\bar{V}$ is velocity, ρ is density, and μ is viscosity.

When Re is less than 2000 and the fluid is homogeneous, streamline flow prevails, but above Re = 3000, turbulent flow occurs. Blood in straight tubes flows in streamlines up to Re = 800 for tubes 2000 μ or less in diameter (Charm et al., 1968). For blood suspensions, Re = $D\bar{V}\rho/K^2$, where K^2 is the square of the Casson viscosity.

Turbulence has been noted in heterogeneous fluids of other suspensions, such as small rubber discs, when Re is between 700 and 1800 (Muller, 1941). The flow of water marked with methylene blue in S-shaped tubes 0.7 cm in diameter was found to be nonlaminar at Re about 550 (Stebhens, 1959). It is not known at what Re number blood in S-shaped tubes becomes turbulent. Coulter and Pappenheimer (1949) found that turbulence for blood in straight tubes was first detected when Re is between 785 and 1140.

In the presence of a branch, the critical Reynolds number for flowing water ranges from 58 to 89% of that in straight tubes 3 mm in diameter (Krovetz, 1963). Branch angle has little effect on the critical Reynolds number. Laminar flow in prebranch tubes or vessels becomes turbulent after it has passed junctions.

Turbulent flow is of importance only under limited circumstances in the microcirculation. For arteries less than 1 mm, Reynolds numbers are extremely low and the flow has few or no oscillations. Thus turbulence might be expected to occur in arteries greater than 3 mm in diameter but not in those less than 1 mm. For example, blood (viscosity 0.035 P) flowing at 10 ml/sec (or 10% cardiac output) in a vessel 0.3 cm in diameter would have a velocity of $10/\pi(0.15)^2 = 140$ cm/sec. The Re would be $(0.3)(140)(1.05)/0.035 = 1260$. Since this result is greater than 800, the flow would be turbulent. It has been suggested that flow in the coronary arteries (vessels larger than those associated with the microcirculation) is likely turbulent, as opposed to the laminar pattern in the other arteries, and this may enhance the tendency to thrombosis.

3.13   SIGNIFICANCE OF REYNOLDS NUMBER IN BLOOD FLOW

With Newtonian fluids, the Reynolds number is a critical parameter for expressing dynamic similarity. A Newtonian fluid flowing in two geometrically similar vessels (same L/D) that have different diameters or lengths, will display the same velocity profile if both tubes have the same Reynolds number. Geometric similarity is a prerequisite for dynamic similarity. In addition, for red cell suspensions, the group $C/\bar{V}^2 \rho$ must also be constant if dynamic similarity is to be achieved.

When blood behaves as a homogeneous Newtonian fluid, the Reynolds number also expresses dynamic similarity when geometric similarity exists. As previously noted, blood behaves as a Newtonian fluid when $C/\bar{V}^2 \rho < 5 \times 10^{-4}$, ϕ is greater than 0.40, and diameter is greater than 155 μ.

It is also possible to express geometric similarity in red cell systems in which radial cell distributions exist. In order to have geometric similarity, there must be similarity in radial cell distribution or in δ/D. As a first approximation, the radial cell distribution can be expressed in terms of a marginal layer width. If δ/D and L/D are constant in different systems, geometric similarity exists and the Reynolds number will again express dynamic similarity (providing K^2 expresses the viscometry of the suspension). This condition exists as long as $C/\bar{V}^2 \rho < 5 \times 10^{-4}$ (Charm and Kurland, 1966). A plot of limiting values δ/D calculated as a function of hematocrit from pressure—flow-rate measurements appears in Fig. 3.6 (see Example 3.3).

3.14   ENERGY REQUIRED FOR CIRCULATION

It has been shown how the frictional pressure loss for blood flowing through a vessel can be calculated (see Table 3.7, Sections 3.5 and 3.6, and Examples 3.1a and 3.1b).

By dividing the frictional pressure loss by the density of blood, the frictional energy loss $(\Delta P)_f/\rho$ is found. If this is examined dimensionally, ΔP_f is in terms of dynes/cm^2 and ρ is designated by g (mass)/cm^2. Thus

$$\frac{\Delta P_f}{\rho} = \text{dynes/cm}^2 \times \text{cm}^3/\text{g(mass)} = \text{dyne-cm/g(mass)}.\frac{(\Delta P)_f}{\rho}$$

is the energy loss per gram (mass) of flowing fluid.

PADDINGTON
COLLEGE LIBRARY.
25, PADDINGTON GREEN,
LONDON, W.2.

However, this is only one of the energy losses experienced by flowing blood. To determine the total energy required to maintain the circulation, we must consider the kinetic, potential, and flow energies, as well as the frictional energy losses.

The energy expended and the blood flow through the circulatory system are related for isothermal systems through the mechanical energy balance. The mechanical energy equation can be expressed by considering the mechanical energy entering and leaving a section of the circulatory system. Let us examine the system defined by the dotted lines in Fig. 3.12. Since the system is assumed to be in a steady state, the energy entering it must equal the energy that leaves. On the basis of 1 g of mass of blood flowing, we have

(3.20)   ENERGY ENTERING

potential + flow energy + kinetic energy + work (heart)

$$gX_1 \quad + \quad \frac{P_1}{\rho} \quad + \quad \frac{\overline{V}_1{}^2}{\lambda} \quad + W =$$

ENERGY LEAVING

$$gX_2 \quad + \quad \frac{P_2}{\rho} \quad + \quad \frac{\overline{V}_2{}^2}{\lambda} \quad + \frac{\Delta P_f}{\rho}$$

where ΔP_f = pressure loss due to friction
λ = 1 for streamline flow; 2 for turbulent flow
X_2, X_1 = height of points 2 and 1, respectively, above a datum plane
g = gravitational constant 980.8 dynes/sec^2

The potential energy entering is gX_1. The units of energy terms must be force-distance/g (mass). To convert height X_1 to an energy term, it must be a force term. Recalling that force is mass times acceleration, and taking the basis of our system as 1 g mass, then $(1)X(g)$ is the force that a gram mass experiences as it is raised through a distance X_1. Thus the potential energy associated with the gram mass after this quantity has been raised is $(1)g(X)$, where g is the gravitational constant.

The kinetic energy entering the system term is $\overline{V}_1{}^2$, which is expressed in terms of force-distance/g if the units of $\overline{V}^2$ are properly arranged. For example, if V is in terms of centimeters per second, $\overline{V}^2$ = cm^2/sec^2 = (cm)(cm)/sec^2. Now centimeters per squared second has the units of acceleration, as does g. Recalling that the basis is 1 gram mass then (1) $(\overline{V}_1{}^2)$ is not just velocity squared but is kinetic energy and the units are gram-centimeters times centimeters per squared second, (cm)(g · cm/sec^2). The term g-cm/sec^2 is a force term, and cm · g-cm/(sec^2) is force-distance − an energy term. The λ, a dimensionless constant for kinetic energy, is 1 for laminar flow and 2 for turbulent flow.

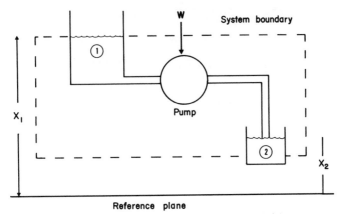

Fig. 3.12 Pumping system defined by broken line.

The work term W is an energy term expressing the energy added to the circulating system by pumping elements such as heart muscle. The frictional work $\Delta P_f/\rho$ represents an energy expenditure and leaves the system in the form of heat. It is assumed the system is isothermal. The total energy balance equation is discussed in more detail in elementary books on fluid flow (e.g., Brown, 1960).

Equation 3.20 contains within it Bernoulli's equation, which indicates the relation between pressure and velocity, but omits frictional loss, potential energy, and work.

To study the circulatory system in terms of a simple flow system (see Figs. 3.13 and 3.14), we can find the useful heart work required for the maintenance of circulation by considering an energy balance taken around the heart. The inlet pressure is P_1 and the outlet pressure is P_2. From equation 3.20 we have

$$(3.21) \qquad \frac{\overline{V}_1^{\,2}}{\lambda} + \frac{P_1}{\rho} + W = \frac{P_2}{\rho} + \frac{\overline{V}_2^{\,2}}{\lambda}$$

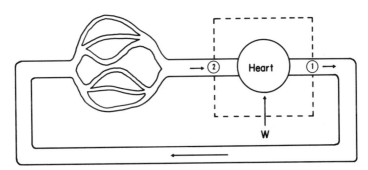

Fig. 3.13 Energy balance with the heart as the system.

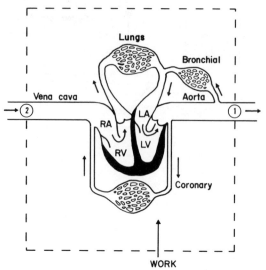

Fig. 3.14   The heart-lung system.

We assume that there is negligible frictional loss in the heart compared with the microcirculation; therefore, $\Delta P_f/\rho = 0$. A convenient basis for equation 3.21 is 1 g of flowing blood. Thus the work W is the work per gram of blood. Rearranging equation 3.21 gives

$$(3.22)\quad W = \frac{1}{\rho}(P_2 - P_1) + \frac{\overline{V}_2{}^2 - \overline{V}_1{}^2}{\lambda}$$

Not only is $P_2 - P_1$ the pressure differential developed by the pump (heart), but it is also the pressure drop through the circulatory system. This can be seen if we consider the section outside the dotted lines in Fig. 3.13.

Employing equation 3.20 again, there is no work entering this system, and we write

$$(3.23)\quad \frac{1}{\rho}(P_1 - P_2) = \frac{1}{\lambda}[\overline{V}_2{}^2 - \overline{V}_1{}^2] + \frac{\Delta P_f}{\rho}$$

Since the mass flow rate at each point is in a steady state, we can calculate the velocity at any point from

$$(3.24)\quad W = \overline{V}A\rho = Q\rho$$

where W = mass flow rate
   A = cross-sectional area
   ρ = fluid density
   $\overline{V}$ = mass velocity
   Q = volume flow rate

When the cross-sectional areas at points 1 and 2 are the same, $\overline{V}_2 = \overline{V}_1$, and we have

$$(3.25) \quad \frac{1}{\rho}(P_1 - P_2) = \frac{\Delta P_f}{\rho}$$

Thus the pressure drop $P_1 - P_2$ through this system is due to friction. The more general, unconstrained system is illustrated in Examples 3.4 and 3.5.

3.15 ENTRANCE AND EXIT LOSSES

When a fluid undergoes a sudden contraction or expansion, as in entrance or exit of vessels, a frictional loss is experienced (Perry, 1953). The sudden expansion of a duct of cross-sectional area A_1, where the mean linear velocity is $\overline{V}_1$, into a duct of larger cross-sectional area A_2, where the velocity is $\overline{V}_2$, is accompanied by the frictional loss of energy,

$$F = \frac{(\overline{V}_1 - \overline{V}_2)^2}{\alpha} = \frac{\overline{V}_1{}^2}{\alpha}\left(1 - \frac{A_1}{A_2}\right)^2$$

where F = dyne-cm/g of mass flowing.

At a sudden reduction in the cross-sectional area of a duct, the frictional loss is

$$F = \frac{K\overline{V}_2{}^2}{\alpha}$$

where V_2 = linear velocity in the smaller section

$$K = 0.4(1.25 - A_2/A_1) \quad \text{for} \quad A_2/A_1 < 0.715$$
$$K = 0.75(1 - A_2/A_1) \quad \text{for} \quad A_2/A_1 > 0.715$$

If the entrance is trumpet-shaped or rounded, K has a value of 0.05. In the small vessels of the microcirculation, entrance and exit vessels are usually negligible.

3.16 ENTRANCE LENGTH

Entrance length is the minimum distance needed for the full development of the flow. The energy loss in the entrance region is greater than the loss occurring when laminar flow is fully developed. The value for the inlet length for laminar flow has been suggested by a number of authors:

Goldstein (1938) $Le = 0.057\,R_w$ (Re)
Schlichting (1960) $Le = 0.08\,R_w$ (Re)
Chang and Atabek (1961)   for oscillating flow in arteries, $Le = 0.16\,R_w$ (Re).
Schlichting (1960)   for turbulent flow, $Le = 1.386\,R_w$ (Re)

Within entrance lengths as small as 20 μ, Palmer (1969) found that the axial accumulation of cells occurred to about 15% of the maximum (see Section 3.4). Axial accumulation of dilute cell suspensions (e.g., 30% in a 40-μ tube) is greater than a 40% suspension. This was determined experimentally by measuring the hematocrit from branches at various points along the length of a capillary tube. Axial accumulation is noted in a channel only 25 μ long; that is, in a capillary whose length is shorter than its diameter. Although the presence of this accumulation may represent a wall exclusion or entrance effect, a major part of the axial accumulation in tubes several hundred times longer than the diameter cannot be accounted for by wall exclusion effects alone; moreover, the contribution from axial drift is greater in long channels carrying dilute suspension. These results agree with the theory that increasing gap width is a function of hematocrit as determined from pressure loss calculations (see Fig. 3.6). Axial accumulation in the 40-μ tube increased up to a length of 10,000 μ and then progressively approached a limit (Palmer, 1971). Thus even with entrance lengths 240 times diameter, the flow of dilute suspensions is not stabilized. For flow with a low Reynolds number (less than 1), which is the prevailing situation in microcirculation, the entry length is simply one tube diameter (Lew and Fung, 1969).

Example 3.1

Determine the velocity profile for red cells in serum flowing in a rigid vessel with a diameter 0.0110 cm.

Given

viscosity of serum	= 0.0174 P
flow rate	= 0.000946 cm^2/sec
length	= 1.325 cm
absolute temperature	= 298°K
cell volume fraction	= 0.38
yield stress	= 10^{-6} dyne/cm^2
suspension density	= 1.05 dynes/cm^2

Solution

(*a*) *Radial cell distribution.* To determine whether a radial distribution exists, $C/\overline{V}^2 \rho$ is evaluated (see Section 3.5). In this case $\overline{V} = 0.000946/\pi(5.5 \times 10^{-3})^2 = 0.1$ cm/sec and $C/V^2\, \rho = 10^{-6}/V(1.05) = 9.5 \times 10^{-5}$. Since $C/V^2\, \rho$ is less than 5×10^{-4}, a radial cell distribution exists.

First the cell distribution must be established (see Section 3.4). The constant A for $\phi = 0.38$ is 0.1593 (see Fig. 3.7). The thickness for each streamline is selected such that $R_w/\Delta R$ is a whole number and ΔR is approximately 4 μ. In this case, $R_w = 0.0055$ cm and, selecting 14 streamlines, $0.0055/14 =$ 0.000392 cm $= \Delta R$.

Using equation A3.8, the flow rate and cell volume fraction for each laminae can be found. In this case, P is not known. It is necessary to assume a value of P until one is found such that $\Sigma \Delta Q_N$ is 0.000946 cm/sec.

As a starting point, the initial P can be taken from Poiseuille's equation:

$$0.000946 = \frac{P}{1.325} \frac{\pi}{8K^2} (5.5 \times 10^{-3})^4$$

where K^2 is found from equation 2.9: $0.0174/[1 - \alpha(0.38)]$, and α is found from equation 2.5 or Fig. 2.9. Thus we have

$$\alpha = 0.07 \exp \left\{ 2.49 \, (0.38) + \frac{1107}{298} \exp \, [-1.65 \, (0.38)] \right\} = 1.3$$

$K^2 = 0.0345$ P

$P = 380,000$ dynes/cm^2

Knowing the initial P, it is possible to calculate the cell volume fraction for each streamline from $N = 1$ to $N = 14$. When ϕ_N has been determined, the viscosity $K_N{}^2$ for each streamline can be found. It then becomes possible to calculate the velocity and flow rate ΔQ_N of each streamline using equations A3.4 and A3.6.

Once each streamline flow rate is known, all such rates can be summed and compared with the given flow rate. In this trial they do not agree. If they do not compare well, another value of P is selected and another trial calculation made. This procedure is carried out until the sum of the streamline flow rates or $\Sigma_{N=1}^{14} \Delta Q_N$ equals the given flow rate of $Q = 0.00946$ cm^3/sec.

The computer program in Section A3.3, Fig. A3.1, is used for this calculation. When P is 116,850 dynes/cm^2, Q is 0.00946. This is the correct value of P. The radial cell distribution found simultaneously is seen in Fig. 3.4, along with the apparent viscosity distribution.

It is interesting to note that when Poiseuille's equation, which assumes a uniform distribution of cells and a parabolic velocity profile, is employed in the foregoing computations, the calculated pressure loss due to friction is 380,000 dynes/cm^2, as compared with 116,850 dynes/cm^2 when the non-uniform cell distribution is considered.

The velocity profile using equation A3.4 is found in Fig. 3.15.

Solution

(b) *Using marginal layer model.* We use equation 3.10 to find P, with δ/D selected from Fig. 3.6 as 1.45×10^{-2} or $\delta = 1.6 \times 10^{-4}$ cm. This is about the

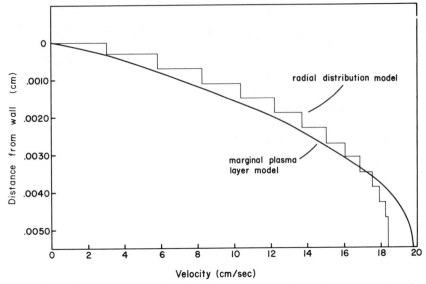

Fig. 3.15   Velocity profile in tube calculated from various flow models; see Example 3.1.

average of the possible range. A computer program for this calculation appears in Section A3.3, Fig. A3.2.

Thus using equation 3.10, $P = 114,000$ dynes/cm². The pressure loss by the marginal layer model agrees within 3% with the pressure loss by the radial cell distribution model. This agreement is within the limits of the computer program. When P has been determined, the point velocity profile is derived using equations 3.16 and 3.17.

Figure 3.15 compares velocity profiles made by both methods. For the sake of this comparison, a pressure loss P of 116,850 dynes/cm² was selected for both methods. Near the center, the radial distribution model has a somewhat blunter profile than the marginal layer model; however, agreement at all points is close.

Example 3.2

In a vessel 0.0200 cm in diameter and 2.00 cm long, the pressure drop is 196 dynes/cm². The cell suspension flowing in the vessel has a cell volume fraction of $\phi = 0.32$ and a limiting apparent viscosity of $K^2 = 0.0202$ P. The density is 1.05 g/cm³ and the yield stress of the blood is 0.12 dynes/cm². Determine the velocity profile and flow rate for the blood in this vessel.

Solution

The flow rate is not known in this case. However, the pressure drop appears to be relatively low, suggesting a low flow rate. As a first approximation, it is assumed that $C/\overline{V}^2\rho$ is greater than 10^{-2} (see Section 3.5). It will be possible to check this assumption after the flow is calculated. If this assumption holds, there is no marginal plasma layer (see Section 3.5) and no radial distribution of cells (see Section 3.4). Equation 3.3 can be used to calculate the velocity profile. At the point where the distance from the center is 0.0040 cm, the velocity is

$$v_{(R=4.0\times10^{-3})} = \frac{1}{0.0202}\left[\frac{196}{(4)(2)}(6.02)^2 - (4.0\times10^{-3})^2\right]$$

$$-\frac{4}{3}\left[\frac{196\times0.12}{(2)(2)}\right]^{1/2}[(0.02)^{3/2} - (4.0\times10^{-3})^{3/2}]$$

$$+0.12[(0.02) - (4.0\times10^{-3})]$$

and

$$v_{(R=4.0\times10^{-3})} = 0.149 \text{ cm/sec}$$

Similarly, the velocity is calculated for other points and the velocity profile is plotted in Fig. 3.2. The check the assumption originally made that $C/\overline{V}^2\rho$ is greater than 10^{-2}, the flow rate is calculated from equation 3.6 and mass average velocity from equation 3.7. In this case δ/D is assumed to be zero (see (see Section 3.4). Equation 3.3 can be used to calculate the velocity profile. At the point, where the distance from the center is 0.0040 cm, the velocity is

The values of the various terms in equation 3.6 are

First term   = 0.00015 cm^3/sec
Second term   = 0.00024 cm^3/sec
Third term   = 0.000047 cm^3/sec
Fourth term   = 0.00000027 (plug) cm^3/sec

The mass average velocity is

$$\overline{V} = \frac{4.4\times10^{-4}}{\pi(2\times10^{-2})^2} = 0.35 \text{ cm/sec} \qquad \text{and} \qquad \frac{C}{\overline{V}^2\rho} = \frac{0.12}{(12.2\times10^{-2})(1.05)}$$

$$= 0.94 \text{ cm/sec}.$$

Thus we were correct in assuming that $C/\overline{V}^2\rho$ is greater than 10^{-2} and δ/D is zero.

Example 3.3

What conditions in a 1000-μ tube would be dynamically similar to the flow conditions in a 110-μ vessel of Example 3.1?

Solution

To be dynamically similar, two vessels must be L/D, $C/\overline{V}^2\rho$, $DV\rho/K_1^2$ or Re and δ/D.

In Example 3.1, $L/D = 1.325/(1.10 \times 10^{-2})$, $DV\rho/K_1{}^2 = 3.29$, $\delta/D = 0.0145$, and $C/\overline{V}^2\rho = 5 \times 10^{-4}$. (As long as $C/\overline{V}^2\rho$ is less than 5×10^{-4}, the term can be dropped from consideration.) It is possible to have $\delta/D = 0.0145$ in a 1000-μ vessel with $\phi = 0.35$ (see Fig. 3.6).

To determine $K_1{}^2$, it is first necessary to find the value of ϕ_1.

From the known Reynolds number of Example 3.1 and noting that

$$Re = \frac{(0.1000\,[Q/\pi(0.5)^2]\,(1.05)}{0.0174/(1 - \alpha\phi_1)} = 3.29$$

for conditions in Example 3.1, we use equation 3.14 as follows:

$$\frac{\phi_1}{0.35} = \frac{1 + 16 \times 10^{-4}}{(0.96)\,2[(0.04) + (0.96)]\,(1 - \alpha\phi_1)}$$

The term $(1 - \alpha\phi_1) = \mu_\rho/K_1{}^2$, and the order of magnitude of $1/K^2$ is $1/0.03$. Thus we have $\phi_1/0.35 \cong 1$.

The viscosity or $K_1{}^2$ is found from equation 2.9:

$$K_1{}^2 = \frac{0.0174}{1 - \alpha\,(0.35)}$$

and

$$\alpha = 0.07 \exp\left\{2.49\,(0.35) + 3.71\,[\exp -1.65\,(0.35)]\right\}$$

$$K_1{}^2 = \frac{0.0174}{1 - (0.34)\,(0.35)} = 0.033\ \text{P}$$

Now solving for Q from the Reynolds number Re, $Q = 0.00810\ \text{cm}^3/\text{sec}$. Thus the conditions for dynamic similarity in the $1000\ \mu$ vessel with the $110\ \mu$ vessel in Example 3.7 are

$Q = 0.00810\ \text{cm}^3/\text{sec}$
$\phi = 0.35$
$L = 12\ \text{cm}$

Under these conditions, the velocity profile in the $1000\ \mu$ vessel will be the same as in the $110\ \mu$ vessel. The dimensionless groups in equation 3.10 are also the same; that is, $D\overline{V}\rho/K_1{}^2$, $PD/\overline{V}^2\rho L$, $C_1/\overline{V}^2\rho$ (in this case negligible), and δ/D.

Example 3.4

Considering the system enclosed by the dotted lines in Fig. 3.14, determine the energy required by the heart for maintaining circulation. The bronchial flow is considered to be negligible.

Given

P_1	$= 10$ mm Hg or $10 \times 1.33 \times 10^3$ dynes/cm^2
P_2	$= 100$ mm Hg $= 1.33 \times 10^5$ dynes/cm^2
Q	$= 6$ L/min $= 100$ cm^3/sec
R_1	$= 1.6$ cm, $K^2 = 0.04$ P
R_2	$= 1.3$ cm

Solution

The frictional loss for flow through the heart is negligible. Employing equation 3.20 and selecting a basis of 1 cm^3 of flowing blood, we write

$$W + \frac{1}{1.05}(1.33 \times 10^4) + X_1 + \frac{\overline{V_1}^2}{\lambda} = \frac{1}{1.05}(1.33 \times 10^5) + X_2 + \frac{\overline{V_2}^2}{\lambda} + \frac{\Delta P_f}{\rho}$$

energy in = energy out

Since points 1 and 2 are at the same level, $X_1 = X_2$, and since frictional effects are negligible $\Delta P_f/\rho = 0$. The average velocity at 1 is $100 = \pi(1.6)^2\,\overline{V}_1$, $\overline{V}_1 = 16.7$ cm/sec. In addition,

$$\overline{V}_2 = \frac{100}{\pi(1.3)^2} = 18.8 \quad \text{cm/sec}$$

and λ is 1 for streamline flow and 2 for turbulent flow, depending on the value of the Reynolds number (see Section 3.12).

At point 1

$$\frac{DV\rho}{K^2} = \frac{(1.6)(16.7)(1.05)}{4 \times 10^{-2}} = 700.$$

At point 2

$$\frac{DV\rho}{K^2} = 790.$$

Since the Reynolds number indicates laminar flow, $\lambda = 1$ and $W = 1/1.05$ $(1.33 \times 10^5 - 1.33 \times 10^4) + (18.8)^2/1 - (16.7)^2/1$

$W = 12.65 + 73 = 85.65$ dyne-cm/g

There is 100 cm^3/sec or 105 g/sec flowing. Therefore, the work/sec or power required for circulation is $85.65 \times 105 = 9000$ dyne-cm/sec.

Example 3.5

Determine the pressure loss for a red cell suspension flowing through the tapered tube shown in Fig. 3.9. The tube is vertical, with the wider section at the top and the red cell suspension flowing down.

Given

flow rate $= 15.58 \times 10^{-4}$ cm^3
plasma viscosity $= 0.0130$ P, reservoir cell concentration, $\phi = 0.20$
tube length $= 6.5$ cm
D_1 $= 0.026$ cm
D_2 $= 0.0078$ cm
ρ $= 1.05$ g/cm^3

Solution

There is no work in this system, and the pressure difference can be found from:

$$1\,(P_1 - P_2) = \frac{V_2{}^2}{\lambda_2} - \frac{V_1{}^2}{\lambda_1} + \Delta P_f/\rho + (X_2 - X_1)\,g$$

To determine λ at sections 1 and 2, the Reynolds number at these sections must be ascertained ($\lambda = 1$ for streamline flow and 2 for turbulent flow). The cell suspension limiting apparent viscosity K^2 is calculated before the Reynolds number is evaluated.
Evaluating,

$$\frac{\overline{V_2}{}^2}{\lambda_2} - \frac{\overline{V_1}{}^2}{\lambda_2} + g\,(X_2 - X_1)$$

and from equation 2.9, we find that

$$K^2 = \frac{0.0130}{1 - \alpha\,(0.20)}$$

$$\alpha = 0.07 \exp\left\{2.49\,(0.2) + \frac{1107}{297}\exp[-1.65\,(0.2)]\right\} = 1.645$$

$$K^2 = 0.0194 \text{ P}$$

Although there is a marginal layer and $\delta/D = 0.05$ (from Fig. 3.6) at the entrance, the effect of this factor on the Reynolds number will be small and can be neglected.
The Reynolds number at (1) is $(0.026)\,(2.9)\,(1.05)/0.0194 = 412$. Therefore flow is streamline, $\overline{V_1}{}^2/\lambda = (2.9)^2$, and

$$gX_1 = (6.5)\,(980.8), \qquad V_2 = \frac{15.58 \times 10}{\dfrac{\pi}{4}\,(7.8 \times 10^{-3})^2} = 32.8 \text{ cm/sec}$$

The Reynolds No. at (2):

$$\frac{D\overline{V}\rho}{K^2} = \frac{(0.0078)(32.8)(1.05)}{0.0194} = 135 \qquad \text{(streamline flow, hence } \lambda = 1)$$

$$\frac{V_2{}^2}{\lambda} = (32.8)^2 \ (\text{cm/sec})^2$$

$$gX_2 = (980.8)(0) = 0$$

The nonuniform tapered vessel is divided into cylindrical segments, as in Fig. 3.9, and each segment is treated as a straight tube. Applying equation 3.10 to finding the pressure drop in each segment, we must also use Fig. 3.6 to find the gap associated with each segment. The yield stress of blood C for $\phi = 0.2$ is about 0.008 dyne/cm^2. The estimated value of $C/\overline{V}^2\rho$ for the first segment is $0.008/(2.9)^2(1.05) \cong 8 \times 10^{-4}$. Since this is greater than 5×10^{-4}, we employ equation 3.10 to determine the gap width in the first section. The true value of $C/\overline{V}^2\rho$ will actually be greater than 5×10^{-4}, since there is a marginal layer and since ϕ, the cell concentration in the central core, will be greater than 0.2.

In order to solve for the actual concentration in the cell core of the first segment, determine marginal layer width using equation 3.15 and Fig. 3.6. Equation 3.14 is then employed to calculate the core cell concentration.

In this case the widest taper has the least influence on the overall pressure drop; also, the marginal layer is less than maximum. Using equation 3.15, we find that the gap width is $\log 8 \times 10^{-4} = (\delta/D)/0.035 \ (\log 5 \times 10^{-2}) + \log 10^{-2}$; δ/D for the first section is 0.033.

Since velocities are greater as the section diameters become smaller, $C/\overline{V}^2\rho$ quickly becomes less than 5×10^{-4} and we can assume that the maximum plasma layer width is developed in all other sections. Thus Fig. 3.6 can serve in determining δ/D for the remaining sections.

Knowing the gap width and the flow rate for each section, it is possible to calculate pressure loss ΔP_f for each section using the lengths designated in Fig. 3.9 in conjunction with equation 3.10.

The sum of the individual pressure losses is the pressure loss due to friction ΔP_f. In this case, $\Delta P_f = 566, 570$ dynes/cm^2.

From Section 3.15 it can be seen that the entrance and exit losses are negligible compared with the frictional loss. Substituting these values in equation 3.20, we find the pressure drop across the nonuniform vessel $P_1 - P_2$.

$$\frac{1}{1.05}(P_1 - P_2) = (1075 - 8.45) + (0 - 6360) + \frac{556,570}{1.05}$$

$$P_1 - P_2 = 567,000 \ \text{dynes/cm}^2$$

It can be seen that potential and kinetic energy effects have a relatively small effect on the total pressure in this case. Experimental values compared with calculated values for several flow rates are listed in Table 3.7.

Example 3.6

A vessel 1 cm long tapers from a diameter of 100 to 50 μ. Blood flowing in the vessel has a yield stress of $C = 0.1$ dyne/cm^2. At what pressure difference across the vessel will flow stop?

Solution

When the wall shear stress is equal to the yield stress, the shear stress at every point in the vessel will be less than the yield stress; thus flow ceases.

The shear stress at the wall τ_w is given by equation 3.1, and we write

$$\tau_w = C = \frac{PR}{L2} = 0.1 = \frac{P(25 \times 10^{-4})}{(1)(2)}$$

$$P = 80 \text{ dynes/cm}^2$$

Example 3.7

Determine the flow rate and hematocrit in the branching system shown in Fig. 3.16.

Given

P_1	$= 16 \times 10^4$ dynes/cm^2
L_A	$= 1.325$ cm
L_B, L_C, L_D	$= 0.700$ cm
ϕ_A	$= 0.38$
Q_A	$= 0.000950$ cm^3/sec
μ_p	$= 0.0174$ P
T_{abs}	$= 298°K$
D_A, D_B, D_C, D_D	$= 0.0110$ cm

Solution

(a) *Solving for* $P_1 - P_2$, ϕ_N, Q_N. Employing the procedure given in Section 3.5, P_2 is determined and the radial distribution of cells is found. This work has been performed in Example 3.1. The radial cell distribution for this case is plotted in Fig. 3.4. The computer program for this calculation is given in Section A3.3, Fig. A3.1. The flow rate for each streamline ΔQ_N (see Appendix equations A3.5 to A3.8) is determined simultaneously with ϕ_N (see Example 3.1). The pressure drop in the lead vessel is found from Example 3.1 to be 116,850 dynes/cm^2 (see Fig. 3.16).

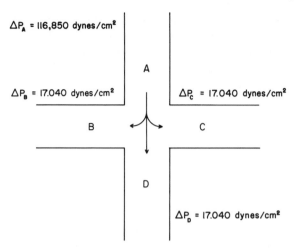

Fig. 3.16   Diagram for branch tube calculation. Calculated results for branches *A, B, C*, and *D* (see Example 3.7) are as follows: Q_A = 0.0095 cm³/sec, $Q_c = Q_B$ = 0.323 x 10^{-3} cm³/sec, Q_D = 0.304 x 10^{-3} ϕ_A = 0.38, $\phi_c = \phi_B$ = 0.373, ϕ_D = 0.394.

(*b*) *Determination of flow rate and cell volume fraction for various segments in the lead vessel.* Segments are defined by chords drawn tangent to one of the concentric circles which are ΔR apart (see Fig. 3.11). The segment is numbered by the *N* of the circle to which the chord is tangent. The subscript 1 is used to define the smaller segments making up the larger segment denoted by *N*.

The flow rate associated with a segment is Q_{NB} and the volume fraction associated with a segment is ϕ_{NB}. In this case, Q_{NB} and ϕ_{NB} are calculated for all values of *N* from 1 to 14. (At *N* = 14, the chord divides the cross section such that the flow is one-half and the associated $\phi_N = \phi_{14} = \phi$; see Table 3.8.)

Table 3.8   Flow Rates and Cell Volume Fractions with Corresponding Pressure Drops in Branch *B* and *D* Fractions of Total Flow Entering Branch *B*

N	Q_{NB} (cm³/sec)	Q_{NB} (cm³/sec)	P_B (dynes/cm²)	Q_D (cm³/sec)	ϕ_D	P_D (dynes/cm²)
7	0.143 x 10^{-3}	0.334	7170	0.666 x 10^{-3}	0.400	34,364
8	0.185 x 10^{-3}	0.346	9419	0.583 x 10^{-3}	0.402	30,509
9	0.231 x 10^{-3}	0.356	11975	0.492 x 10^{-3}	0.402	26,216
10	0.279 x 10^{-3}	0.366	14702	0.395 x 10^{-3}	0.400	21,400
11	0.330 x 10^{-3}	0.375	17430	0.294 x 10^{-3}	0.391	16,290
12	0.381 x 10^{-3}	0.382	20000	0.191 x 10^{-3}	0.371	10,078
13	0.432 x 10^{-3}	0.388	22897	0.891 x 10^{-4}	0.302	7,170
14	0.481 x 10^{-3}	0.392	25316	–	–	–

(c) *Determination of flow rate in branches.* The pressure drop across each branch leading from the intersection must be equal. The flow rate through each of the branches adjusts, rendering the pressure drop equal in each branch.

In Fig. 3.16 the flow rate and the volume fraction in branches B and C are equal. The flow rate in branch D, Q_D, is

$$(3.26) \qquad Q_D = Q_A - 2Q_{NB}$$

and the volume fraction in branch D, ϕ_D is

$$(3.27) \qquad Q_D \phi_D = Q_A \phi_A - 2Q_{NB} \phi_B$$

It is necessary to compute the pressure drop in branch B for the various Q_{NB} and ϕ_{NB} calculated in subsection (b). The procedure is the same as that illustrated in Example 3.1 for finding pressure drop (e.g., see Table 3.8).

The corresponding flow rates and cell volume fractions for branch D are found from equations 3.26 and 3.27. The pressure drop for each flow rate in branch D is determined just as these values calculated for branch B; see Table 3.8.

The condition in the branches that exist when $\Delta P_B = \Delta P_D$ describes the correct flow rate for branches B and D. Table 3.8 indicates that $\Delta P_B = \Delta P_D$ for conditions described between $N = 10$ and $N = 11$. Through interpolation in the table, we see that $\Delta P_B = \Delta P_D = 117{,}040$ dynes/cm^2.

Further interpolation for flow rate and cell volume fraction for this pressure drop gives

$$Q_{NB} = 0.323 \times 10^{-3} \text{ cm}^3/\text{sec} = Q_C$$
$$\phi_{NB} = 0.373 = \phi_C$$
$$Q_D = 0.304 \times 10^{-3} \text{ cm}^3/\text{sec}$$
$$\phi_D = 0.394$$

The conditions for these calculations were taken from the experiments of Gelin (1963). In the following tabulation, we compare calculated results with those of Gelin.

	Gelin Experiment	Calculated
Q_C	0.335×10^{-3} cm^3/sec 0.315×10^{-3} cm^3/sec	0.323×10^{-3} cm^3/sec
ϕ_C	0.37	0.373
Q_D	0.296×10^{-3} cm^3/sec	0.304×10^{-3} cm^3/sec
ϕ_D	0.40	0.394

Clearly, the experimental results agree well with the calculated results.

In the experimental data of Gelin it is noted that pressure at the entrance to lead vessel A is 160,000 dynes/cm^2. However, the pressure drop through each branch is calculated to be 17,040 dynes/cm². Therefore, 27,110 dynes/cm² is unaccounted for, possibly because of a pressure drop at the entrance to the branches. The calculation of flow in the branch assumes that there is no substantial disturbance of the flow pattern as it is developed in the lead vessel.

Since experimental and calculated results are in such good agreement, it may be that although pressure loss occurs at the branch entrance, it does not disturb the flow pattern sufficiently to affect the calculation of cell volume fraction or flow rate. If the cells were completely mixed at the branch entrance, the flow rate and cell volume fraction in each branch would be equal.

APPENDIX   DERIVATION OF CELL DISTRIBUTION AND FLOW RATE EQUATIONS

A3.1   Calculation of Cell Distribution in a Straight Tube

Suppose that the cross section of a cylindrical vessel is divided into annuli, each ΔR thick and each representing a streamline; see Fig. 3.11. Considering incremental changes in velocity Δv from streamline to streamline, the velocity of any streamline N is

(A3.1) $v_N = v_{N-1} + \Delta v_N$

where v_{N-1} is the velocity of the adjacent streamline closer to the vessel wall.

(A3.2) $\dfrac{\Delta v}{\Delta R} = \dfrac{PR}{2LK^2}$

As the streamlines or annuli are numbered, N designates the streamline number and $N = 1$ is next to the streamline annulus vessel wall; N increases toward the center. The distance from the center to any streamline is $R = (R_w - N\Delta R)$. Substituting the longer expression for R, equation A3.2 becomes

(A3.3) $\Delta v_N = \dfrac{P}{2LK_N{}^2} (R_w - N\Delta R)\,\Delta R$

where $K_N{}^2$, the limiting apparent viscosity associated with streamline N (see Chapter 2), is a function of the cell volume fraction related to the streamline as described by equations 2.9 and 2.5.

Since the velocity at the wall is zero, we use equation A3.3 to determine that the velocity of the streamline next to the wall (where $N = 1$) is

$$v_1 = 0 + \dfrac{P}{2LK_1{}^2} (R_w - 1\Delta R)\,\Delta R$$

where $K_N{}^2$ is as described for equation A3.3.

At the streamline, where $N = 2$, the velocity of the streamline is

$$v_2 = \frac{P}{2LK_1{}^2} (R_w - \Delta R) \Delta R + \frac{P}{2K_2{}^2 L} (R_w - 2\Delta R) \Delta R$$

Generally, we can write

$$(A3.4) \quad v_N = \frac{P\Delta R}{2L} \left(\frac{R_w - \Delta R}{K_1{}^2} + \frac{R_w - 2\Delta R}{K_2{}^2} + \cdots + \frac{R_w - N\Delta R}{K_N{}^2} \right)$$

The flow associated with each streamline or annulus is its cross-sectional area times velocity or

$$\Delta Q_N = 2\pi(R_w - N\Delta R)v_N \Delta R$$

and substituting equation A3.4 for v_N, we have

$$(A3.5) \quad \Delta Q_N = 2\pi(R_w - N\Delta R) \left[\frac{P\Delta R}{2L} \frac{(R_w - \Delta R)}{K_1{}^2} + \frac{R_w - 2\Delta R}{K_2{}^2} + \cdots \right.$$

$$\left. + \frac{R_w - N\Delta R}{K_N{}^2} \right]$$

Equation 2.3 indicates that

$$K_1{}^2 = \frac{\mu_P}{1 - \alpha_1 \phi_1}, \qquad K_2{}^2 = \frac{\mu_P}{1 - \alpha_2 \phi_2}, \qquad \text{and} \qquad K_N{}^2 = \frac{\mu_P}{1 - \alpha_N \phi_N}$$

Substituting equation 2.9 for $K_N{}^2$, ΔQ_N becomes

$$(A3.6) \quad \Delta Q_N = \pi(R_w - N\Delta R) \left(\frac{\Delta R^2}{\mu_P} \right) \left(\frac{P}{L} \right) [(R_w - \Delta R)(1 - \alpha_1 \phi_1)$$

$$+ (R_2 - 2\Delta R) 1 - \alpha_2 \phi_2 + \cdots + (R_w - N\Delta R)(1 - \alpha_N \phi_N)]$$

The cell volume fraction ϕ_N associated with each streamline is calculated by substituting in equation 3.9:

$$\sum_{N=1}^{N} \Delta Q_N \quad \text{for} \quad Q_{R_w \to R}$$

Alternatively, the cell volume fraction with any streamline is

$$(A3.7) \quad \phi_N = Q_M + A \left[2 \frac{(\Delta Q_1 + \Delta Q_2 + \cdots + \Delta Q_N)}{Q_T} - 1 \right]$$

where Q_T = total flow rate = $\displaystyle\sum_{N=1}^{R_w/\Delta R} \Delta Q_N$

Substituting for ΔQ, this becomes

(A3.8) $\phi_N = \phi_m + A \left\{ 2\pi \dfrac{(R_w - N\Delta R)}{Q_T} \dfrac{\Delta R^2}{\mu_p} \left(\dfrac{P}{L}\right) [(R_w - \Delta R)(1 - \alpha_1 \phi_1) \right.$

$\left. + (R_w - 2\Delta R)(1 - \alpha_2 \phi_2) + \cdots + (R_w - N\Delta R)(1 - \alpha_N \phi_N)] - 1 \right\}$

In solving for ϕ_N, an initial value of Q_T must first be estimated (e.g., from Poiseuille's equation). For example, having estimated Q_T, ϕ_N is solved for $N = 1$ using equation A3.8. This permits evaluating ΔQ_1 from equation A3.6, and so on. Next ϕ_N is determined for $N = 2$ and ΔQ_2 is evaluated and so on.

The value of Q_T is next compared with $\Sigma_{N=1}^{R_w/\Delta R} \Delta Q_N$. If they do not agree within 1%, the trial-and-error procedure is repeated, using $\Sigma_{N=1}^{R_w/\Delta R} \Delta Q_N$ for the new value of Q_T.

When in two successive trials, values of $\Sigma_{N=1}^{R_w/\Delta R} \Delta Q_N$ agree within 1%, the correct value for total flow rate and the correct cell distribution have been found. If $\Delta P/\Delta L$ is not known but Q_T is, the same type procedure is followed. In this case the initial $\Delta P/\Delta L$ is estimated – possibly from Poiseuille's equation (equation 1.1). Again, values of $\Delta P/\Delta L$ are varied until $\Sigma_{N=1}^{R_w/\Delta R} \Delta Q_N$ agrees with the known Q_T.

The sum of the flow rates of all streamlines must equal the total flow rate, and the following condition must be fulfilled:

(A3.9) $Q_T = \displaystyle\sum_{N=1}^{R_w/\Delta R} \Delta Q_N$

A typical calculation of this kind appears in Example 3.1a. Both $\Delta Q_1 + \Delta Q_2 + \cdots + \Delta Q_N$ and Q_T (equation A3.7) are direct functions of plasma viscosity; therefore, cell distribution is independent of plasma viscosity because plasma viscosity cancels out in the ratio of $\Delta Q_1 + \Delta Q_2 - - - \Delta Q_N/Q_T$.

When $C/\overline{V}^2 \rho$ is between 10^{-2} and 5×10^{-4}, the distribution function A in equation 3.9 becomes A_v and can be calculated from

(A3.10) $\log \dfrac{C}{\overline{V}^2 \rho} = \dfrac{A_v}{A} [\log (5 \times 10^{-2})] + \log 10^{-2}$

where A_v = distribution function when it varies with velocity; this is substituted for A in equation A3.8 when $C/\overline{V}^2 \rho$ is between 10^{-1} and 5×10^{-4}
A = value of A found in Fig. 3.7.

When $C/V^2 \rho$ is greater than 10^{-2}, equations 3.6 or 3.8 are used to calculate flow rate and there is no cell distribution along the radius in this model.

It is interesting to note that even though the streamline at the center has the maximum velocity, the mass flow rate is a maximum at a point about midway between the wall and centerline. The reason for this, of course, is that the mass associated with centerline is very small (see Example 3.1).

The partial annulus contributed by each streamline to the segment making up the cross section of flow entering the branch is found as follows. Total area of an annulus is designated by A_{TN}, where N is the annulus or streamline number ($N = 1$ being next to the wall). The difference between the areas of the two concentric circles making up the annulus is A_{TN}.

(A3.11) $A_{TN} = \pi [(R_w - (N - 1)\,\Delta R)^2 - (R_w - N\,\Delta R)^2]$

The area of the partial annulus is found by subtracting the area of two consecutive segments formed by a chord as it intersects the concentric circles forming the annuli (e.g., chord BB' in Fig. 3.11).

The partial annulus area is designated as A_N, and A_{Ni} is the area of the segment formed by the chord tangent to the circle designated by i and intersecting circle N (e.g., see chord BB' in Fig. 3.11).

The area of partial annulus N is

(A3.12) $A_N = A_{(N-1)i} - A_{(N)i}$

Area of partial annulus $N = 1$ (the cross-hatched area) in Fig. 3.11 formed by chord BB' is

$A_1 = A_{0,2} - A_{1,2}$

The area of segment $A_{(N)i}$ is

(A3.13) $A_{(N)i} = (R_w - N\Delta R)^2 \sin^{-1} [(R_w + N\Delta R)^2 - (R_w - i\Delta R)^2]^{1/2}$
$- (R_w - i\Delta R)[(R_w - N\Delta R)^2 - (R_w - i\Delta R)^2]^{1/2}$

The flow rate associated with a part of a streamline making up the flow that enters a branch is proportional to the partial area of the streamline (i.e., A_N) and is designated by Q_{NB}:

(A3.14) $\Delta Q_{NB} = \dfrac{A_N}{A_{TN}} \Delta Q_N$

The area contribution of the smallest segment making up the large segment entering branch would be as a segment designated $A_{(i-1)(i)}$. All the other streamline contributions are in the form of a partial annulus.

The total flow rate associated with the segment representing cross section of flow entering the branch and with a chord tangent at $N = i$ is

(A3.15) $Q_{NB} = \displaystyle\sum_{N=1}^{N-1} \dfrac{A_N}{A_{TN}} \Delta Q_N + \dfrac{A_{(i-1)(i)}}{A_{Ti}} \Delta Q_i$

The cell volume fraction associated with the branch flow or segment flow is

$$(A3.16) \quad \phi_{NB} = \frac{\sum\limits_{N=1}^{N-1} A_N/A_{TN} \, \Delta Q_N \phi_N + [A_{(i-1)}(i)]/A_{Ti} \, \Delta Q_i \phi_i}{Q_{NB}}$$

where ϕ is the cell volume fraction associated with streamline i.

From equations A3.15 and A3.16, the relationship between Q_{NB} and Q_{NB} can be calculated.

For a given flow Q_{NB} entering the branch, the flow continuing downstream is

$$(A3.17) \quad Q_T - Q_{NB} = Q_D$$

where Q_T = flow rate entering main vessel
Q_D = flow rate in main vessel after branch

The cell volume fraction after the branch associated with Q_D is

$$(A3.18) \quad Q\phi - Q_{NB} \, \phi_{NB} = Q_D \, \phi_D, \quad \text{see example 3.7}$$

A3.2   Complete Flow Rate Equation in the Presence of a Marginal Layer

In the presence of a marginal layer and an unsheared plug of cells in the central region of a tube (see Fig. 3.8a) the complete flow rate equation is given by

$$(A3.19) \quad \bar{V} = \frac{P}{L}\left(\frac{R_c}{R_w}\right)^2 R_c^2 \left\{ \frac{1}{K_1^2} \left[\frac{1}{8} - \frac{1}{2}\left(\frac{R_P}{R_c}\right)^2 + \frac{1}{4}\left(\frac{R_P}{R_c}\right)^4 \right] \right.$$

$$- \frac{4}{3}\left(\frac{R_P}{R_c}\right)^{1/2} \frac{1}{K_1^2}\left[\frac{3}{14} - \frac{R_P}{R_c}\frac{1}{R_c^2} - \frac{2}{7}\left(\frac{R_P}{R_c}\right)^{7/2} \right] + \frac{R_P}{R_c}$$

$$\frac{1}{K_1^2}\left[\frac{1}{6} - \frac{1}{2}\left(\frac{R_P}{R_c}\right)^2 + \frac{1}{3}\left(\frac{R_P}{R_c}\right)^3 \right] + \frac{1}{4\mu_p}\left[\frac{1}{2}\left(\frac{R_w}{R_c}\right)^4 \right.$$

$$- \left(\frac{R_w}{R_c}\right)^2 + \frac{1}{2} \right] + \frac{1}{K_1^2}\left(\frac{R_P}{R_c}\right)^2 \left[\frac{1}{4}\left(1 - \left(\frac{R_P}{R_c}\right)^2\right) - \frac{2}{3}\left(\frac{R_P}{R_c}\right)^{1/2} \right.$$

$$\left. \left. \left(1 - \left(\frac{R_P}{R_c}\right)^2 + \frac{1}{2}\frac{R_P}{R_c}\left(1 - \frac{R_P}{R_c}\right) + \frac{1}{4}\left(\frac{R_P}{R_c}\right)^2\left(\frac{R_w}{R_c}\right)^2 - 1\right) \right] \right\}$$

where μ_P = plasma viscosity

$\overline{V}$ = mass average velocity

R_c = radius of cell core including plug

R_P = radius of plug of unsheared cells = $2LC_1/P$

P/L = pressure/length

C_1 = cell core yield stress

R_w = tube radius

$K_1{}^2$ = cell core Casson viscosity, or asymptotic apparent viscosity of cell core.

This equation assumes laminar flow. When conditions are such that marginal layers do not exist, $R_c = R_w$.

Equation A3.19 is derived in accordance with the following steps. First the velocity profile in each of the three regions is found:

(A3.20)   IN THE MARGINAL PLASMA LAYER

$$\frac{P}{2\mu_P L} \int_R^{R_w} R \, dR = \int_v^0 dv$$

$$v = \frac{P}{4\mu_P L} [R_w{}^2 - R^2]$$

(A3.21)   FLOW RATE IN THE PLASMA GAP

$$Q_P = 2\pi \int_{R_c}^{R_w} R v \, dR$$

Equation A3.20 is substituted for v. Similarly, in the annular section of sheared cells, the point velocity is given by equation 3.16.

The flow rate in the sheared core of cells is

$$Q_s = 2\pi \int_{R_P}^{R_c} R v \, dR$$

where equation 3.16 is substituted for v.

The velocity or the plug is the same as the point velocity at the edge of the sheared cell section (where $R = R_P$).

The flow rate of the plug is

$$Q_{P_1} = \pi R_P{}^2 \, v_{P_1}$$

The total flow rate is

$$Q = Q_P + Q_s + Q_{P_1}$$

The mass average velocity is

$$\overline{V} = \frac{Q}{\pi R_w{}^2}$$

A3.3   Computer Programs Used for Chapter 3

```
C       DR. CHARM - RADIAL CELL DISTRIBUTION
        COMMON QTOTAL,RW
        DIMENSION PHIN(50),FPHIN(50),DELV(50),VN(50),DELQ(50),QN(50)
       1,PS(50)
        DIMENSION ATN(50),DELWNB(50),QNBP(50)
        DIMENSION QNB(50),PHINB(50)
        READ (1,1000) P,XL,RW,K,PHM,XMU,TAU
  1000 FORMAT (3F7.2,I2,3F7.4)
        PHMX=PHM
        DELTAR=RW/K
C           SET INITIAL 3 VALUES AND PRINT
        CALL FORDTE (A1,A2)
        DO 510 IZ=1,20
     1 WRITE (3,1100) A1,A2,RW,K,DELTAR,P,XL,PHM,XMU,TAU
  1100 FORMAT (10H1DR. CHARM,100X,2A4//1X,3HRW=,F9.4,4H   K=,I2,10H  DELTA
       1 R=,F7.5,4H   P=,F9.1,4H   L=,F9.3,6H  PHI=,F9.2,5H  MU=,F9.4,
      26H  TAU=,F9.2//)
        WRITE (3,1110)
  1110 FORMAT (37H RADIAL CELL DISTRIBUTION COMPUTATION//)
        IK=K+1
        DELV(1)=0.
        VN(1)=0.
        DELQ(1)=0.
        PHIN(1)=PHM-A(PHM)
        ALPHA=.07*EXP(2.49*PHM+((1107./(273.+T AU))*EXP(-1.65*PHM)))
        QTOTAL=(3.14157*P*RW**4)/((8.*XMU*XL)/(1.-ALPHA*PHM))
        FPHIN(1)=F(PHIN(1),TAU,XMU)
        J=1
        WRITE (3,1200) J,PHIN(1),FPHIN(1)
  1200 FORMAT (5X,2HJ=,I3,3X,4HPHI=,E12.4,3X,7HF(PHI)=,E12.4)
C           NOW ITERATE FOR REST OF PHIS AND QTOTAL
        DO 500 IX=1,20
C
        DO 401 N=2,IK
        PH=.1
        RN=RW-(N-1)*DELTAR
C
        DO 300 I=1,20
        DELV(N)=(P/(2.*XL))*((RN*DELTAR)/F(PH,TAU,XMU))
        VN(N)=0.
        DO 200 J=1,N
   200 VN(N)=VN(N)+DELV(J)
        DELQ(N)=2.*3.14157*RN*VN(N)*DELTAR
        QN(N)=0.
        DO 150 J=1,N
   150 QN(N)=QN(N)+DELQ(J)
```

```
      PHIN(N)=PHM+A(PHM)*((2.*QN(N))/QTOTAL-1.)
      EP=ABS((PHIN(N)-PH)/PH)
      IF (EP-.01) 400,400,300
  300 PH=PHIN(N)
  400 FPHIN(N)=F(PHIN(N),TAU,XMU)
      WRITE (3,1200) N,PHIN(N),FPHIN(N)
  401 WRITE (3,1300) RN,DELV(N),VN(N),DELQ(N),QN(N)
 1300 FORMAT (10X,3HRN=,F9.5,6X,5HDELV=,E12.4,6X,3HVN=,E12.4,
     16X,5HDELQ=,E12.4,6X,3HQN=,E12.4)
      EP=ABS((QTOTAL-QN(IK))/QTOTAL)
      WRITE (3,1600) IX,QTOTAL,QN(IK),EP
 1600 FORMAT (1H0,I26,3E14.5)
      IF (EP-.01) 600,600,500
  500 QTOTAL=QN(IK)
  600 IF (ABS(QTOTAL-.000946)/QTOTAL-.01) 102,102,505
  505 IF (QTOTAL-.0009553) 506,506,507
  506 P=P+.07*P
      GO TO 510
  507 P=P-.05*P
  510 CONTINUE
  102 WRITE (3,1500)
 1500 FORMAT (10H CONVERGED)
      QX=QTOTAL
      PX=P
C         NOW COMPUTE FLOW RATE IN BRANCH
      WRITE (3,1100) A1,A2,KW,K,DELTAR,P,XL,PHM,XMU,TAU
      WRITE (3,2000)
 2000 FORMAT (32HONEW COMPUTE FLOW RATE IN BRANCH//)
      IKX=IK-1
      DO 710 I=1,IKX
      FLOW=0.
      QP=0.
      XI=RW-I*DELTAR
      DO 715 J=1,I
      XJ=RW-(J-1)*DELTAR
      XJP=XJ-DELTAR
      IF (I-IKX) 720,721,720
  721 RF=.5
      GO TO 722
  720 RF=(ASEG(XI,XJ)-ASEG(XI,XJP))/(3.14159*(XJ**2-XJP**2))
  722 FLOW=FLOW+RF*DELQ(J+1)
  715 QP=QP+(RF*DELQ(J+1)*PHIN(J+1))
      QNBP(I)=QP
      QNB(I)=FLOW
  710 PHINB (I)=QNBP(I)/QNB(I)
C            FLOW RATE
      WRITE (3,2200)
 2200 FORMAT (///)
      DO 723 N=1,IKX
  723 WRITE (3,2300) N,QNBP(N),QNB(N),PHINB(N)
 2300 FORMAT (3H N=,I3,11H   QNBP(N)=,E12.5,10H    QNB(N)=,E12.5,
     112H    PHINB(N)=,E12.5)
      P2=20000.
      XL=.7
      DO 890 ICY=1,2
      DO 890 N=1,K
      GO TO (901,902),ICY
  902 QNSPNS=(QX*PHMX)/2.-QNBP(N)
      QNS=QX/2.-QNB(N)
      PNS=QNSPNS/QNS
      QNB(N)=2.*QNS
      PHM=PNS
      GO TO 903
  901 PHM=PHINB(N)
  903 ALPHA=.07*EXP(2.49*PHM+((1107./(273.+T AU))*EXP(-1.69*PHM)))
      QTOTAL=(3.14157*P*RW**4)/((8.*XMU*XL)/(1.-ALPHA*PHM))
      P=20000.
      WRITE (3,3000) A1,A2,KW,K,DELTAR,XL,PHM,XMU,TAU,P
```

```
3000 FORMAT (48H1DR, CHARM - FINAL BRANCH FLOW RATE COMPUTATIONS,54X,
     12A4//6H    RW=,F7.4,4H  K=,I2,9H  CELTAR=,F7.5,10H  BRANCH LENGTH=,
     2F6.3,7H  PHIM=,F6,4,5H  MU=,F7.4,6H  TAU=,F5.2//6H  P2=,F10.4//
     38X,74HN       PHINB       QNB     SGMT      P        PHIN        Q
     4N     LDIFF)
     WRITE (3,3100) N,PHINB(N),QNB(N)
3100 FORMAT (I9,F1C.4,E14.4)
     DO 888 IJ=1,2C
     RN=RW-(N-1)*DELTAR
     DO 886 IX=1,2C
     DO 885 I=1,K
     RX=RW-(I-1)*DELTAR
     PH=.01
     DO 880 J=1,20
     DELV(I)=(P/(2.*XL))*((RX*DELTAR)/F(PH,TAU,XMU))
     VN(I)=0.
     DO 801 II=1,I
 801 VN(I)=VN(I)+DELV(II)
     DELQ(I)=2.*3.14157*RX*VN(I)*DELTAR
     QN(I)=0.
     DO 802 II=1,I
 802 QN(I)=QN(I)+DELQ(II)
     PHIN(I)=PHM*A(PHM)*((2.*QN(I))/QTLTAL-1.)
     EP=ABS((PHIN(I)-PH)/PH)
     IF (EP-.01) 885,885,880
 880 PH=PHIN(I)
 885 CONTINUE
     EP=ABS((QTOTAL-QN(K))/QTOTAL)
     IF (EP-.01) 887,887,886
 886 OTOTAL=QN(K)
 887 EP1=ABS((QNB(N)-QN(K))/QNB(N))
     IF (EP1-.01) 891,891,889
 889 IF (QN(K)-QNB(N))806,806,807
 806 P=P+.07*P
     IF (P-PX) 888,888,811
 807 P=P-.05*P
     IF (P) 811,811,888
 888 CONTINUE
 811 WRITE (3,3300) EP1
3300 FORMAT (20X,31HDID NOT CONVERGE - DIFFERENCE =,E12.4)
 891 DO 892 I=1,K
 892 WRITE (3,3200) I,P,PHIN(I),QN(I)
3200 FORMAT (33X,I5,F11.2,E12.4,E12.4,E13.4)
 890 CONTINUE
     CALL EXIT
     END


     FUNCTION A(PHI)
     COMMON QTLTAL,RW
     IF (PHI) 10,10,20
 10  A=0
     RETURN
 20  IF (PHI-.27) 30,30,40
 30  A=EXP(.673057*ALOG(PHI)-1.09834)
     GO TO 25
 40  IF (PHI-.30) 50,60,60
 50  A=.197333*PHI+.0848001
     GO TO 25
 60  A=.70821435*PHI-.7607145*PHI**2
 25  V=QTOTAL/(3.14159*RW**2)
     PSI=.1/(V**2*1.05)
     IF (PSI-5.E-4) 21,21,22
 21  RETURN
 22  IF (PSI-1.E-2) 23,10,10
 23  A=(A*(ALOG10(PSI)-ALOG10(1.E-2)))/(ALOG10(5.E-2))
     RETURN
     END
```

```
      FUNCTION ASEG(XI,XJ)
      COMMON QTOTAL,RW
      IF (XI-XJ) 5,10,10
   10 ASEG=0.
      RETURN
    5 XX=SQRT(XJ**2-XI**2)
      ASEG=(XJ**2)*ATAN((XX/XJ)/(SQRT(1.-(XX/XJ)**2)))-
     1XI*SQRT(XJ**2-XI**2)
      RETURN
      END


      FUNCTION F(PHI,TAU,XMU)
      COMMON QTOTAL,RW
      IF (PHI) 10,10,20
   10 F=0.
      RETURN
   20 ALPHA=.07*EXP(2.49*PHI+((1107./(273.+TAU))*EXP(-1.65*PHI)))
      F=XMU/(1.-ALPHA*PHI)
      RETURN
      END
```

Fig. A3.1 *Definitions:* P = pressure; XL = length; K = no of annuli or streamlines, PHM = ϕ_m; XMU = μ_p, TAU = T temperature. DELTAR = ΔR = streamline thickness RW = vessel Radius (see Examples 3.1 and 3.7)

```
    C     MARGINAL LAYER PROGRAM S.CHARM
          REAL MU,L,K1SQ
          READ (1,1000) MU,W,L,I,PHI,F,C,RHO,DEL,D
     1000 FORMAT(F5.4,F7.6,F5.3,F3.0,F4.3,F4.3,F2.1,F4.2,F6.5,F5.4)
          RW=D/2.
          P=(8*C*MU*L)/((3.1416)*RW**4)
          N=1
       10 QG=(3.1416)*(P/(2.*MU*L))*((RW**2/2.)-(RW-DEL)**2/2.)**2
          Q1=Q-QG
          PHI1=C*PHI/Q1
          ALPHA=.07*EXP(2.49*PHI1+(1107/T)*EXP(-1.65*PHI1))
          K1SQ=MU/(1-ALPHA*PHI1)
          C1=F*PHI1
          VBAR=C/((3.1416)*RW**2)
          Z1=32.*K1SQ/(C*VBAR*RHO)
          Z2=((P*D)/(VBAR**2*RHU*L))*((1-(1-2*DEL/D)**4)/(1-ALPHA*PHI1)+
         X(1-2*CFL/L)**4)+(C1/((VBAR**2)*RHL))*((1-2*DEL/D)**3*((16./3.)-(32
         X./7.)*(((P*D)/(C1*L))*(1-2*DEL/D))**.5))
          FP=ABS((Z1-Z2)/Z1)
          WRITE(3,1100) P,QG,Z1,Z2, PHI1,K1SQ,Q1,C1,MU,Q,L,T,PHI,F,C,RHO
     1100 FORMAT(1X,8E12.4/4X,8E12.4//)
          IF (FP-.01)5,5,15
        5 CALL EXIT
       15 IF (Z1-Z2) 20,20,25
       20 P=P-.05*P
          GU TO 30
       25 P=P+.07*P
       30 IF (N-50)35,40,40
       35 N=N+1
          GU TO 10
       40 WRITE(3,1200)
     1200 FORMAT (17H,DID NOT CONVERGE)
          CALL EXIT
          END
```

Fig. A3.2 *Definitions:* MU = μ_p; Q = flow rate; L = length; T = absolute temperature; PHI = ϕ = cell fraction; P = pressure drop; C = yield stress; RHO = ρ; DEL = δ = gap width; D = diameter. (See equation 3.10)

```
C     FLOW RATE WIYH YIELD STRESS  S.CHARM
      REAL L,KSW
      READ (1,1000) P,KSQ,L,RW,C
1000  FORMAT (F4.0,F5.4,F4.2,F5.4,F3.2)
      Q1=((22/7.)*P/(4*KSQ*L))* ((RW**2)/(2)-.5*(((2*L*C)/(P))**2))
      Q2=(R*22/(7.*3.*KSQ))*(((P*C)/(2*L))**.5)*(((RW**3.5)/(2))-
     X((RW**3.5)/(2))*((2*L*C/(P))**2)-(2/7.)*((RW**3.5)-((2*L*C/(P))**
     X3.5)) )
      Q3=(2*(22/7.)*C/(KSQ))* ((RW**3/(2.))-(RW/2.)*((2*L*C)/(P)
     X)**2)-(((RW**3)/(3.)-(((2*L*C)/(P))**3)/(3.)))) )
      Q4=(1/KSC)*((P/(4*L))*(RW**2-((2*L*C)/(P))**2)-(4/3.)*((
     XP*C/L)**.5)*((RW**1.5)-((2*L*C/P)**1.5))+C*(RW-(2*L*C/P))*
     X((2*L*C/P)**2)*22/7.)
      QT=Q1+Q2+Q3+Q4
      GU TO 15
15    WRITE (3,1100) QT,Q1,Q2,Q3,Q4
1100  FORMAT(1X,2E15.4)
      CALL EXIT
      END
```

Fig. A3.3 *Definitions:* P = pressure drop; L = length; KSQ = K^2 = apparent viscosity (limiting) or Casson viscosity squared; RW = vessel radius; C = yield stress. (See equation 3.6)

```
C     VELOCITY DISTRIB, W/YIELD STREESS S, CHARM
      REAL L,KSW
      READ (1,1000) P,KSQ,L,RW,C
1000  FORMAT (F4.0,F5.4, F4.2, F5.4,F3.2)
      RI=0
      DO 10 I=1,26
      V=(1/KSQ)*((P/(4*L))*(RW**2-RI**2)-(4/3.)*((P*C/(2*L))**.5)*
     X((RW**1.5)-(RI**1.5))+C*(RW-RI))
      GO TO 15
15    WRITE (3,1100) V,RI
1100  FORMAT ( 1X,2E15.4)
10    RI=RI+RW/25
      CALL EXIT
      END
```

Fig. A3.4 *Definitions:* P = pressure drop; L = length; KSQ = K^2; RW = R_w; C = C. (See equation 3.3)

```
C     VELOCITY DISTRIBUTION S.CHARM
      REAL MU,L,K1SQ
      READ(1,1000) P,MU,L,RW,DEL,K1SQ,C1
1000  FORMAT (F7.0,F5.4,F5.3,F5.4,F6.5,F5.4,F3.2)
      RI=0
      DO 10 I=1,26
4     IF (RI-(RW-DEL)) 5,20,20
5     V=(P/(4.*MU*L))*(RW**2-(RW-DEL)**2)+(1/(K1SQ))*((P/(4*L))*((RW-DEL
     X)**2-(RI**2)))
      GO TO 15
20    V=(P/(4*MU*L))*(RW**2-RI**2)
      GO TO 15
15    WRITE (3,1100) V,RI
1100  FORMAT (1X,2E15.4)
10    RI=RI+RW/25.
      CALL EXIT
      END
```

Fig. A3.5 *Definitions:* P = pressure drop; MU = plasma viscosity; L = length; DEL = gap width; K1SQ = $K_1^2 \cong K^2$; C1 = $C_1 \cong C$. [See equation (3.16)]

Flow Through Capillaries

Chapter 4

4.1 THE CAPILLARIES

CAPILLARIES ARE THE SMALLEST UNITS of the circulatory system, the vessels through which mass and heat exchange with tissues and organs occur. It has been noted that about 2% of the plasma flow exchanges with the tissues in passage through capillaries (e.g. Berne and Levy, 1967). A blood flow rate of 6 L/min suggests about 1 cm^3/sec of plasma exchanges with the tissue through the capillary walls.

The average capillary is about 10^{-3} cm in diameter, 0.1 cm long and with a capillary wall one endothelial cell thick (about 1×10^{-4} cm). Capillary surface area in the lung is 5×10^6 to 7×10^6 cm^2 at three-fourths of lung capacity and can be varied through the opening and closing of capillaries.

More than 40% of the capillaries in the left ventricular apical myocardium of rat, cat, and rabbit are between 3 and 4 μ in diameter. Average red cell diameters in these animals are 5.7 μ. Erythrocytes readily pass through capillaries half their diameter (Sobin and Tremer, 1972).

Permeability in the capillaries associated with 100 g of muscle is equivalent to that of a membrane 7000 cm^2 in area, 0.5 μ thick, containing 5×10^{12} pores 40 to 45 Å in radius (Landis and Pappenheimer, 1963). There are about 17 pores/μ^2. Pore area does not exceed 0.1% of endothelium. The shape of pores may be rectangular or cylindrical. A distribution of pores exists, and the pore size differs among various organs (Palade, 1968; Grotte, 1956). It is estimated that there is one large pore (250 to 350 Å in diameter) for every 34,000 small pores (40 Å). Electron microscope studies suggest one geometry of the inter-endothelial cell cleft − namely, about 5000 Å long and about 200 Å wide except over a short length of about 200 Å, where it constricts to about 40 Å (Karnovsky, 1967, 1970).

Three types of capillary have been described − continuous, discontinuous, and fenestrated. In muscle, skin, the central nervous system, lung, and mesentery, the endothelial cells form a continuous layer and are surrounded by a continuous basement membrane. These vessels are referred to as "continuous" capillaries. In the sinusoids of the liver, spleen, and bone marrow, the large gaps that can be seen between the endothelial cells and the basement membrane in these vessels are said to be "discontinuous." In the capillaries of the intestine, renal glomerulus and tubules, endocrine glands, choroid plexus and ciliary body, and the retina mirabilia, the endothelium is thinned in certain special regions to form a single electron-dense layer. These regions have been called fenestra, and the capillaries are said to be of a "fenestrated" type (Michel, 1972).

A detailed study of fenestrated capillaries of the rat indicated that the fenestral regions are circular, having a 40-Å diameter; the membrane or "diaphragm" covering them has a central blob 15 Å in diameter (Clementi and

129

Palade, 1969). It is suggested that the fenestra are formed by the progressive thinning of opposing regions of inner (luminal) and outer cell membranes of endothelium. The only muscle capillaries that have been shown to possess fenestra are those of the external eye muscles (Collin, 1969).

One of the most prominent features of the capillary endothelium is the presence of a large number of circular or oval inclusions of cell membrane called the micropinocytolic vesicles.

Pressure at the proximal arteriolar end of the capillary is about 32 mm Hg, whereas at the distal end it is about 15 mm Hg. Osmotic pressure differences across the capillary wall due to circulating plasma protein and small ions (oncotic pressure) is about 25 mm Hg. The driving force for water transfer through the capillary wall is the sum of the hydrostatic pressure difference and osmotic pressure difference across the capillary wall. The hydrodynamic passage of fluid through pores in the capillary wall is the favored theory for water exchange. As intravascular pressure in the capillary increases, the capillary radius increases, tending to reduce the frictional energy loss of cells and plasma passing through.

4.2 ELASTICITY AND STRESS IN CAPILLARY WALLS

Vessels of the circulatory system are not rigid; rather, they respond to changes in internal pressure with changes in diameter. The vessel property that governs these changes is elasticity. In larger vessels of the microcirculation (e.g., small arteries, arterioles, venules, and veins), vessel wall diameter is principally responsive to nervous control, rather than transmural pressure and wall elasticity. In capillaries, however, diameter is not subject to nervous control.

LaPlace's equation is frequently employed to express the relationship between pressure and radius and cylindrical vessels.

$$(4.1) \quad t = P_t R_a$$

where t = tension force/length
P_t = transmural pressure difference
R_a = vessel radius

Although it is a convenient expression, LaPlace's equation does not consider the thickness of the vessel wall and thus omits an important parameter from consideration. The properties of vessel wall material that actually determine the relationship between transmural pressure and vessel radius are the elastic modulus E_w and the Poisson ratio v. The thickness of the vessel wall plays an important role in setting the relationship between vessel diameter and pressure.

The elasticity of any material is expressed in terms of the elongation of a bar of the material under a given stress or per unit area. The simplest relationship between elongation and stress is given by equation 4.2, which is known as Hooke's law:

(4.2) $S = E_w e$

where e = strain
        S = stress
        E_w = elastic modulus

The strain e is the fractional elongation of an element; that is, $\Delta L/L$ where ΔL is the change in the length of the material with length L. The stress or force/unit area acting in the wall of a thin cylindrical vessel under pressure is (see Fig. 4.1)

(4.3) $S = \dfrac{P_t R_a}{T}$

where T = thickness
        P_t = pressure differential across cylinder wall or transmural pressure
        R_a = radius of cylinder

The strain in this case is $\Delta R/R_a$. This is the same ratio as the change in the length of circumference (i.e., $2\pi dR_a$) to the length of circumference or $2R_a$ at a section in the vessel or $2\pi \Delta R_a/2\pi R_a = \Delta R_a/R_a$. The wall thickness T varies with the change in radius. The relationship between T and R_a is given by

(4.4) $\dfrac{dT}{T} = -\nu \dfrac{dR_a}{R_a}$

or

$$\frac{T}{T_0} = \frac{(R_a)^{-\nu}}{R_0}$$

where: ν = Poisson ratio for material or vessel wall
         T_0 = thickness of wall at "rest" radius R_0
         R_0 = ν cylinder rest radius or radius with zero transmural pressure
         R_a = cylinder radius with transmural pressure difference P_t

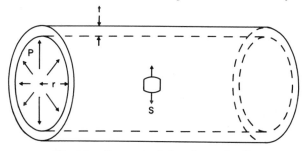

Fig. 4.1   Pressure and stress in vessel wall.

The Poisson ratio v is (unit lateral contraction)/(unit axial elongation), considering a bar of material. For materials that have the same elastic properties in all dimensions (isotropic materials), $v = 0.25$.

We can assume for small changes in radius that the vessel wall acts as a Hookian material, and the relationship between transmural pressure in the vessel and the vessel radius is

(4.5) $$\frac{R_a}{R_0} = \frac{P_t R_0}{E_w T_0} \left(\frac{R_a}{R_0}\right)^v + 1$$

In a vessel filled with flowing blood, the pressure decreases as the flow proceeds downstream; the radius as influenced by transmural pressure also decreases (as expressed by equation 4.5). The shape a vessel assumes depends on the hydrostatic and osmotic pressure differences along its length and on its elastic properties. Knowing the transmural pressure along the vessel, it is possible to calculate the vessel shape using equation 4.5.

Elastic characteristics of living vessels have not yet been determined experimentally. A complicating factor is that vessels are supported by other structures and tissues. McDonald (1960) has described the elastic modulus of a number of vessels (see Table 4.1). The elastic characteristics of blood vessel walls indicate that they are not simple Hookian material, as suggested by equation 4.2. At strains $\Delta R/R$, corresponding to an increase in size from 5 to 25%, the elastic modulus E_w may increase progressively from a value of 1.2×10^6 to 4.0×10^6 dynes/cm^2 in mesentery vessels 100 to 200 μ in diameter (Wiederhielm, 1965). At strains exceeding 25%, the modulus increases rapidly, reaching a value of 45.5×10^6 dynes/cm^2.

Estimates for the elastic modulus for individual components of the blood vessel wall (i.e., the smooth muscle, the collagen, and the elastic tissue) are as follows (Wiederhielm, 1965):

1. Collagen derived from tendon: 300×10^6 dynes/cm^2.
2. Elastic tissue from ligamentum nuchae: 3×10^6 dynes/cm^2.
3. Relaxed smooth muscle in taenia coli: 0.1×10^6 dynes/cm^2.

Although the elastic modulus of endothelium has never been measured, most investigators agree that endothelial cells are easily deformed. Wiederhielm suggests a value of 0.1×10^6 dynes/cm^2.

From a knowledge of the composition of a vessel wall, it is possible to estimate the elastic modulus for a relaxed vessel wall from the following equation:

(4.6) $E_{(wall)} = E_{(sm)} A_{(sm)} + E_{(coll)} A_{(coll)} + E_{(end)} A_{(end)} + E_{(el)} A_{(el)}$

where $E_{(sm)}, E_{(coll)}, E_{(end)}, E_{(el)}$ = elastic modulus for smooth muscle, collagen, endothelium, and elastic tissue, respectively

$A_{(sm)}, A_{(coll)}, A_{(end)}, A_{(el)}$ = corresponding fractions of the cross-sectional area of the wall

Table 4.1 Elastic Moduli Of Arteries[a]

Tissue	Method of measurement	Young's Modulus (dynes/cm^2 x 10^{-6})	Comments
Ligamentum nuchae	Longitudinal strip	4.6	Calculated by Burton (1954)
Ligamentum nuchae	Longitudinal strip	40	Small extensions
Thoracic aorta	Longitudinal strip	1.24	
Thoracic aorta	Longitudinal strip (dog)		
Thoracic aorta	Longitudinal strip (dog) (static)	3	70% extensions (i.e., "natural" length)
Thoracic aorta	Longitudinal strip (dog) (dynamic)	2–18	Range from 10 to 70% extensions
Thoracic aprta	Longitudinal strip (dog, cow)	1.4	Extensions up to 40%
Thoracic aorta	Whole vessel collagen extracted	3	Calculated by Burton (1954)
Thoracic aorta	Tangential modulus from pulse-wave velocity. (dog)	2.5	Calculated from pulse-wave velocity of about 5000 cm-sec found by Dow and Hamilton (1939), Laszt and Muller (1952a)
Thoracic aorta	Whole vessel (longitudinal) (dog)	2.0–3.0	Extensions from excised length up to 10% greater than "natural" length
Thoracic aorta	Whole vessel (tangential) (static)	3.0	Pressures 20 to 100 mm Hg
Thoracic aorta	(tangential) (static)	20.0	Maximal value found in any specimen at 200 mm Hg
Thoracic aorta	(tangential) (static)	1.2	At 40 mm Hg (mean of 10 specimens)
Thoracic aorta	(tangential) (static)	4.4	At 100 mm Hg (mean of 10 specimens)
Thoracic aorta	(tangential) (static)	16.1	At 200 mm Hg (mean of 10 specimens)
Thoracic aorta	(tangential) (dynamic)	4.7	2.0 cm/sec 100 mm Hg (mean of 10 specimens)
Thoracic aorta	(tangential) (dynamic)	5.3	18.0 cm/sec 100 mm Hg (mean of 4 specimens)

[a]From McDonald (1960).

In the constricted blood vessel wall, Wiederhielm refers to the "viscosity" of the vessel wall to describe its behavior as a function of strain. A vessel that had been constricted with a topical application of epinephrine was subjected to internal pressure. The vessel dilated abruptly at first and subsequently, along a more prolonged time course, exhibited a behavior similar to creep in plastic material. This indicates that the viscosity characteristics of the vascular smooth muscle cells increased greatly in the process of contraction. The elastic modulus of the wall also increased in vasoconstriction from 8.1×10^6 to 23.2×10^6 dynes/cm^2. Thus vasoconstriction is associated with an increase in both elastic and viscous moduli, resulting in a stiffening of the elastic wall. The response of living vessels to pressure differs from vessels in dead animals, living vessels being more elastic (Kurland et al., 1966).

Arterial walls of fresh excised human and canine arteries behave as nonlinear homogeneous compressible material and can be described by six elastic moduli for each of the three principal directions (Tichner and Sacks, 1967). For various internal pressures ranging from 50 to 300 mm Hg, the elastic modulus varied from about 2×10^6 to 30×10^6 dynes/cm^2, and the Poisson ratio varied between about 0.2 and 0.7 for the three principal directions. Computations of elastic modulus are inadequate for biological systems except within a narrow range. For calculation purposes, wanting a better model, we assume that vessel walls behave as Hookian material, over small stress ranges (see Section 4.5).

4.3   CAPILLARY SHAPE DUE TO TRANSMURAL PRESSURE

We know from equation 4.5 that the capillary radius varies with transmural pressure. As hydrostatic or osmotic pressure change, the shape of the vessel changes (see Fig. 4.2).

The compression stress due to transmural pressure may close the vessel when hydrostatic pressure is sufficiently low. To calculate decreases in radius due to compression, P_t is negative in equation 4.5. For example, to reduce R_a to $R_a/R_0 = 0.2$ or $R_a = 1 \times 10^{-4}$ cm, the P_t required can be estimated by assuming the following values:

$E_w = 10^6$ dynes/cm^2, $\nu = 0.25$, $T_0 = 1 \times 10^{-4}$ cm, from equation 4.5

$$0.2 = \frac{P_t(10^{-4})(0.2)^{1/4}}{10^6 \ (10^{-4})} + 1$$

or

$$P_t = -1.2 \times 10^6 \text{ dynes/cm}^2$$

However, it is impossible to obtain so great a transmural pressure acting to

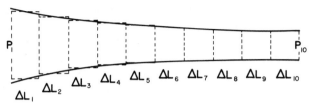

Fig. 4.2 Theoretical shape of capillary with elastic wall. For calculation purposes the length is divided into 10 increments. For calculated change in radius of capillary as a function of length for conditions, see Example 4.1.

compress the capillary, for the following reason. A transmural pressure of such magnitude is greater than the oncotic pressure (i.e., osmotic pressure influenced by protein), which is available in a capillary to produce compressive pressure. Oncotic pressure is 3.33×10^4 dynes/cm^2 or less. Also closing must occur in a manner not described by equation 4.5, which is based on a gradual change. The compressive stress closing the capillary must perform that function by overcoming the compressive strength of the capillary wall – an "elastic closing" will not do.

The cytoplasm in the endothelial cells composing the capillary wall is probably in gel form rather than fluid to offer support to the capillary wall against transmural pressure (Fung, 1966). For the capillary to close, it appears that the gel structure may become a sol at some critical stress and revert back to gel when the stress is removed. It is also concluded that capillaries of the rabbit mesentery are almost entirely supported by the surrounding tissue (Fung and Zweifach, 1966). Capillary distensibility is of no physiological significance, being less than 0.08% mm Hg (Burton, 1966). However, capillary shape could influence flow resistance and flow rate, and this factor should be considered in the analysis of capillary flow; see Section 4.7 and Example 4.1.

Precapillary arterioles frequently show no change in lumen for pressure changes and behave as though they were rigid. This has been referred to as the "flat top" effect (Baez, 1968). It is not certain that this effect occurs in capillaries. In some arterioles an autoregulatory response has been observed whereby the micro vessel contracts on pressure rise and dilates on pressure drop (Bayliss concept). In arterioles and possibly in capillaries, therefore, calculated passive responses to transmural pressure do not always apply. The "flat top" effect may be explained by inelastic wall components predominating under certain conditions, whereas the elastic components predominate in others (Burton, 1965).

4.4 ANALYSIS OF FLOW IN CAPILLARIES

Viscosity is not a relevant property of blood when blood flow in capillaries is being studied. Blood does not flow as a homogeneous suspension in capillaries as it does in larger vessels; rather, it flows as a two-phase system — cells and plasma. Plasma alone is the liquid phase, and plasma viscosity is the significant viscosity parameter. The viscosity of hemoglobin within the cell may influence the elastic properties of the cell, but this is part of the cell elastic characteristics.

Consider a capillary with a radius R_a, which is larger than the rest radius of a cell r_c, by an amount, δ (Fig. 4.3). The cell distorts under pressure, causing an

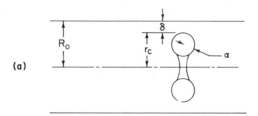

(a)

Fig. 4.3   Cell and vessel at rest.

increase in the gap between the cell and the wall (Fig. 4.4). When the cells are oriented to move downstream in the same position, as in Fig. 4.5, ("stacked flow"), the velocity profile must be a plug flow type, since the entire cell moves with the same velocity as at the cell edge (see Fig. 4.6). The velocity at the cell edge is determined by the velocity of plasma that is undergoing luminar flow between the vessel wall and the edge of the cell. As pressure increases, the cell distorts, shortening the cell radius r_c by an amount Δr. Velocity of the cell is

$$(4.7) \quad v_c = \frac{P}{4\mu_p L} [R_a{}^2 - (r_c - \Delta r)^2]$$

where v_c = velocity of cell
R_a = radius of vessel at given pressure
r_c = rest radius of cell
Δr = change in projected radius of cell due to deformation under pressure
μ_p = plasma viscosity

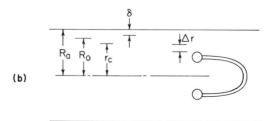

(b)

Fig. 4.4   Capillary with diameter greater than
red cell; cell and vessel under pressure.

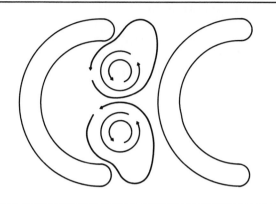

Fig. 4.5   Cells in "stacked flow," showing plasma eddies.

The change in cell radius due to stress distortion is (see Appendix to Chapter 4)

$$(4.8) \quad \Delta r = \frac{3V_0 r_c{}^2}{\pi a^2} \left[\frac{\Delta P/L}{(r_c - \Delta r)^5 \, E_c(1 - \nu_c)^2} \right]^{1/3}$$

$$\cos \left[\frac{1}{2} \left\{ \frac{\Delta P}{E_c L} (r - \Delta r) \, [24(1 - \nu_c)] \right\}^{1/3} \right]$$

where V_0 is cell volume.

The surface area of one face of the cell is

$$(4.9) \quad A_c = \frac{P}{3L} (r_c - \Delta r)^3 \left[\frac{24 \, (1 - \nu_c)}{E_c (P/L)^2 \, (r_c - \Delta r)^2} \right]^{1/3}$$

The flow rate through a capillary slightly larger than the cell is

$$(4.10) \quad Q = \frac{\pi \Delta P}{8\mu_p L} \left[R_a{}^4 - (r_c - \Delta r)^4 \right]$$

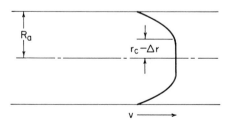

Fig. 4.6   Velocity profile in a capillary.

The radius of the capillary is also a function of pressure, as shown by equation 4.5 (Charm and Nelson, 1967).

In this analysis, the cells were considered to assume a paraboloid or parachute shape under stress. However, it has been suggested that the parachute shape often observed is not an axisymmetric shape as formerly thought but is instead the basic biconcave disc shape of the red cell, with the upstream end flattened by the pressure gradient (Skalak and Branemark, 1969).

The normal biconcave disc shape of the red cell can be stretched 10 to 15% without hemolysis. The biconcave shape is maintained by ATP (LaCelle, 1971).

The force required to deform a normal red cell in saline is estimated by a sedimentation packing procedure to be less than 1.7×10^{-6} dyne (Brooks et al., 1970).

Cells in capillaries may flow in "stacked" flow as described in Fig. 4.5, or the cells may orient "edge on," with the opposite sides of the cell pushed in and the central part of the disc pushed out. The shape is cylindrical, with the leading edge convex and trailing edge concave. This type of orientation occurs at low velocities (0.2 mm/sec) and tube diameters less than cell diameters (Hochmuth et al., 1970).

If a capillary wall is relatively rigid, the cell elastic properties play a major role in determining the character of flow. If the vessel wall is as elastic as the cell, however, the cell properties are less important. Rand (1967) deduced the elastic modulus for the red cell membrane to be 10^6 to 10^8 dynes/cm^2. The flow rate through a capillary has been calculated using equations 4.10 and 4.8 for various conditions; see Example 4.1.

When walls are rigid (e.g., as in a polycarbonate sieve), passage of normal red cells is restricted when the diameter is less than 3 μ. However when the cells are hardened, (e.g., with acetaldehyde), they are unable to pass 6.8-μ pores (Gregersen et al., 1967).

Osmotic pressure of cell contents and plasma affect the cell elastic properties (i.e., E_c, elastic modulus, and ν_c, Poisson ratio). Thus the flow rate through the capillary as represented in equation 4.7 is influenced by osmotic pressure difference across the cell.

Since the capillary radius R_a varies along the length of capillary, it may be necessary to calculate the effect of capillary taper on flow rate. As a rule, the taper is such that radii at the capillary do not vary more than 10% (see Table 4.2). The capillary length is divided into increments ΔL (Fig. 4.2), and the flow rate and pressure drop associated with each increment are calculated. The following procedure is used to calculate flow rate through capillaries.

1. *Calculate R_a.* Suppose that we know ν_c, Ec, r_0, T_0, r_c, E_w, ν, L, entrance pressure P_1, exit pressure, P_{10}, osmotic pressure difference across wall, and ΔL. For the first section assume a value of $\Delta P_1/\Delta L$ and determine P_t for section 1: $P_1 - \Delta P_{osmotic} = P_t$. The initial assumed value for $\Delta P_1/\Delta L$ can be estimated from $(P_1 - P_{10})/L$.

Table 4.2   Radius and Pressure Drop as a Function of Distance in a Non-rigid Capillary[a]

	Radius (cm)	Distance along Capillary (cm)	ΔP (dynes/cm^2)
1	5.26×10^{-4}	0.01	1.98×10^3
2	5.20×10^{-4}	0.02	2.09×10^3
3	5.14×10^{-4}	0.03	2.21×10^3
4	5.08×10^{-4}	0.04	2.34×10^3
5	5.02×10^{-4}	0.05	2.48×10^3
6	4.96×10^{-4}	0.06	2.62×10^3
7	4.90×10^{-4}	0.07	2.78×10^3
8	4.83×10^{-4}	0.08	2.95×10^3
9	4.77×10^{-4}	0.09	3.13×10^3
10	4.71×10^{-4}	0.10	3.33×10^3

[a]See Example 4.1.

2. *Calculate Q.* Using the assumed value $\Delta P_1/\Delta L$ and value of R_a from step 1, Q is calculated using equations 4.8 and 4.10. The value of Q remains constant in all sections (transfer of water across capillary wall is neglected here).

3. *Calculate P_2, R_{a_2} and $\Delta P_2/\Delta L$.* Determine P_2 from $\Delta P_1/\Delta L$ ($P_2 = P_1 + \Delta P$) and calculate R_{a_2} for second sections using equation 4.5. Knowing Q, ΔP_2 is calculated using equations (4.8) and (4.10).

4. *Compare sum of ΔP with $P_{10} - P_1$.* The ΔP for all sections is calculated in a manner similar to step 3, and the sum of ΔP is compared with $P_1 - P_{10}$. When these two values agree, the correct $\Delta P_1/\Delta L$ is assumed. When they do not agree, new values of $\Delta P_1/\Delta L$ are assumed until agreement is reached.

This procedure is illustrated in Example 4.1. The computer program for this calculation appears in Section A4.3. For examples of how the various parameters involved in capillary flow affect flow rate, see Tables 4.3 to 4.5. It is revealed that the elastic modulus of the wall E_w, and wall thickness T_0 can be varied; but as long as the product of these values is constant, they do not affect flow rate.

Table 4.3   Effect of Pressure on Flow Rate[a]

Entrance P (dynes/cm^2)	ν_c	E_w (dynes/cm^2)	T_0 (cm)	E_c (dynes/cm^2)	ν_c	Q (cm^3/sec)
0.426×10^5	0.25	0.1×10^7	0.1×10^3	0.5×10^8	0.5	0.60×10^{-6}
0.6×10^5	0.25	0.1×10^7	0.1×10^3	0.5×10^8	0.5	0.96×10^{-6}

[a]Increase in pressure causes a linear increase in flow rate.

Table 4.4   Effect of Varying Cell and Wall Elastic Properties

ν	E_w (dynes/cm^2)	T_0(cm)	E_c (dynes/cm^2)	ν_c	Q(cm^3/sec)
Group 1[a]					
0.25	0.1×10^7	0.1×10^{-3}	0.5×10^8	0.5	0.40×10^{-6}
0.25	0.1×10^7	0.1×10^{-3}	0.5×10^8	0.3	0.37×10^{-6}
0.5	0.1×10^7	0.1×10^{-3}	0.5×10^8	0.3	0.37×10^{-6}
Group 2[b]					
0.25	0.1×10^7	0.1×10^{-3}	0.5×10^8	0.3	0.37×10^{-6}
0.25	0.1×10^8	0.1×10^{-3}	0.5×10^8	0.3	0.37×10^{-6}
0.25	0.1×10^7	0.1×10^{-3}	0.5×10^9	0.3	0.32×10^{-6}
Group 3[c]					
0.25	0.1×10^7	0.1×10^{-3}	0.5×10^8	0.3	0.37×10^{-6}
0.25	0.1×10^7	0.1×10^{-2}	0.5×10^8	0.3	0.37×10^{-6}

[a] 1.7 x change in cell Poisson ratio or wall Poisson ratio has little effect on flow rate.
[b] 10 x change in cell or wall elastic modulus has little effect on flow rate.
[c] 10 x change in wall thickness has no effect on flow rate.

With pressure remaining constant, flow is decreased slightly by increasing the elastic modulus times wall thickness, (E_wT_0), or by making the wall stiffer. Increasing the cell Poisson ratio slightly serves to increase flow. Upon doubling the Poisson ratio of the vessel wall, the flow rate is slightly decreased (see Table 4.4). Table 4.5 indicates that the flow rate is proportional to the plasma viscosity, other things being constant. It is interesting to note that a change in plasma viscosity from 0.013 to 0.02 P, which is not uncommon in certain diseases, reduces capillary flow rate by nearly 50%. The change in radius along the capillary is relatively small for any of these changes. The foregoing procedure did not take into account the transmural passage of water along the length of the capillary under the influence of osmotic and hydrostatic pressure.

Fung (1966) has suggested that capillaries are more rigid than larger vessels. Even by employing the same order of magnitude of elastic modulus for capillaries that was measured for larger vessels, however, it appears that there is still little change in radius along the capillary. For a given entrance pressure over the range of parameter changes noted in Table 4.4, the change in radius along the capillary length is about 10% (see Table 4.2). A 40% increase in pressure is calculated to result in about a 40% cause increase in flow rate in capillaries (see Table 4.3). The property having the greatest influence on capillary flow rate or pressure drop is plasma viscosity.

An estimate of flow rate in capillaries can be obtained by assuming a viscosity of 0.02 P and applying Poiseuille's equation (Prothero and Burton, 1962). Using

Table 4.5 Calculated Effect of Plasma Viscosity on Flow Rate through Capillary[a]

ν	E_w (dynes/cm²)	T_0 (cm)	V_c (cm³)	r_c (cm)	E_c (dynes/cm²)	ν_c	P_1, (Entrance) (dynes/cm²)	P_{10}, (Exit) (dynes/cm²)	μ_p (P)	Q (cm³/sec)
0.25	0.1×10^7	0.1×10^{-3}	0.84×10^{-10}	0.4×10^{-3}	0.5×10^8	0.3	0.416×10^5	0.200×10^5	0.013	0.37×10^{-6}
0.25	0.1×10^7	0.1×10^{-3}	0.84×10^{-10}	0.4×10^{-3}	0.5×10^8	0.3	0.416×10^5	0.200×10^5	0.015	0.32×10^{-6}
0.25	0.1×10^7	0.1×10^{-3}	0.84×10^{-10}	0.4×10^{-3}	0.5×10^8	0.3	0.416×10^5	0.200×10^5	0.020	0.24×10^{-6}

[a] Capillary length = 0.1 cm; $R_w = 5 \times 10^{-4}$.

Prothero and Burton's estimation, the flow rate through the capillary in Example 4.1 is 2.40×10^{-7} cm^3/sec, as compared with 3.7×10^{-7} cm^3/sec calculated with a consideration of cell and wall properties (i.e., equation 4.8). There is about a 35% difference between these two calculated results. Significantly, a flow rate of this order of magnitude results in a wall shear rate of about 5000 sec^{-1} and a wall shear stress of 50 to 100 dynes/cm^2. We can use the data in Table 4.2 and Poiseuille's equation to calculate that the apparent viscosity at the entrance section to the capillary is 0.0156 P, whereas at the exit it is 0.033 P, with an average of about 0.025 P through the length of the capillary. The elegant Prothero-Burton calculation gives a useful estimate of flow rate, as compared with the relatively lengthy calculation employing elastic properties of cells and walls. However, the more lengthy calculation is helpful in analyzing details of flow in capillaries.

Equations for calculating pressure drops in capillaries have been developed through experimenting with flexible red cell models later filled with silicone oil in large tubes and applying dimensional analysis to the experimental data (Lee and Fung, 1969; Sutera et al., 1970). (see Fig. 4.7).

The total pressure drop is calculated by considering the pressure drop for plasma alone in the capillary (Sutera et al):

$$(4.11) \quad \Delta P_{\text{Pois}} = 32 \frac{\mu_p \overline{V}}{D_T} \cdot \frac{L}{D_T}$$

and adding the pressure drop associated with the cells:

$$\Delta P_{\text{cells}} = \phi \overline{V} \frac{\pi D_T^2}{4} \frac{L}{v_c} \frac{1}{V_0} \frac{\Delta P^*}{\mu_p \overline{V}/D_T} \frac{\mu_p \overline{V}}{D_T}$$

The total pressure drop in the capillary is $\Delta P_{\text{pois}} + \Delta P_{\text{cells}}$. Moreover, from Fig. 4.7 we know that

$$\frac{\Delta P^*}{\mu_p \overline{V}/D_T} \quad \text{is a function of} \quad \frac{\mu_p \overline{V}}{E_c D_T}$$

where μ_p = plasma viscosity
$\quad D_T$ = tube diameter
$\quad \Delta P^*$ = pressure drop for single cell
$\quad n$ = number of cells in capillary
$\quad E_c$ = elastic modulus of the cell
$\quad \overline{V}$ = average mass velocity
$\quad v_c$ = cell velocity
$\quad \phi$ = volume fraction of cells in blood

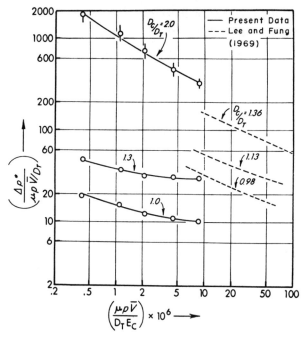

Fig. 4.7　Pressure loss for single cell in capillary ΔP^* as function of cell strain. Dotted lines results from Lew and Fong, 1969 (from Sutera et al., 1970), with the permission of Academic Press and the authors.

It is possible to solve Example 4.1 for capillary pressure loss using two methods. The two calculation methods result in the same answer, although their approaches are quite different – even to the extent of requiring different properties. They agree, however, because the overwhelming pressure loss effect is due to plasma flow. Essentially the same pressure loss can be calculated by simply applying Poiseuille's equation to plasma flow in the capillary, neglecting the red cell entirely, as well as wall elasticity; see Example 4.1b.

4.5　CONCENTRATION OF CELLS IN CAPILLARY

The concentration fraction of cells associated in the core of the capillary can be found by noting that cell flow rate in the feed ($Q\phi$), must equal the cell flow rate in the core $Q\phi$. Thus

$$(4.12) \qquad Q\phi = Q_c \phi_c$$

The flow rate in the core Q_c is equal to $Q - Q_g$, where Q_g is plasma flow rate in the region surrounding the gap, and

$$(4.13) \quad Q_g = \int_{(r_c - \Delta r)}^{R_a} 2\pi R_v \, dR$$

Plasma flow rate in the annulus surrounding the cells in single file is

$$(4.14) \quad Q_g = \frac{\pi \Delta P}{8 \mu_p L} [R_a - (r_c - \Delta r)^2]^2$$

The flow rate of the cells and plasma between cells also can be found from cell velocity of equation 4.7, in that

$$(4.15) \quad Q_c = \pi(r_c - \Delta r)^2 v_c = \pi(r_c - \Delta r)^2 \frac{\Delta P}{4 \mu_p L} [R_a^2 - (r_c - \Delta r)^2]$$

The volume fraction of cells in the core of the capillary becomes

$$\phi_c = \frac{\phi Q}{Q_c}$$

and

$$(4.16) \quad \phi_c = \frac{\phi}{2} \left[\left(\frac{R_a^2}{r_c - \Delta r} \right)^2 + 1 \right]$$

Equation 4.8 can be used to calculate Δr in equation 4.16.

Whitmore (1967) offered a similar analysis but did not quantitatively consider the effects of cell and capillary wall elastic properties. His analysis is based on the relationship for simple shear in the presence of (a) a marginal layer as developed by Thomas (see equation 3.24) and (b) the continuity equation (equation 3.21). According to his analysis, the minimum possible apparent relative viscosity is obtained when the axial train contains only cells. For a hemotocrit of 40%, the viscosity in a capillary is only about 7% greater than the plasma; in bulk, however, the blood viscosity is about 150 to 200% greater than plasma viscosity. These percentages are in general agreement with Prothero and Burton's experimental result and with the calculated result considering cell and wall elastic properties as noted in Section 4.6 and Example 4.1.

Equation 4.16 reveals that when there is a rigid cell ($\Delta r = 0$) and the cell radius is equal to vessel radius, then $\phi_c = 0$. When the cell vessel wall distorts under pressure such that the flexible cell radius $r_c - \Delta r$ is half the capillary radius, then $R_a/r_c - \Delta r) = 2$ and the volume fraction of cells flowing in the core is $1/2(4 + 1) = 5/2$ that of the feed volume fraction of cells. This is also the condition for maximum core concentration. The maximum core concentration, $\phi_c = 1.0$, is recorded when the core is composed only of cells. This occurs with a hematocrit of 40% or $\phi = 0.4$ when

$$\left[\left(\frac{R_a}{r_c - \Delta r}\right)^2 + 1\right] \frac{0.4}{2} = 1 \qquad \text{or} \qquad \frac{R_a}{r_c - \Delta r} = 2$$

that is, the radius of the distorted cell is half the vessel radius.

If a vessel tapers and the flow proceeds to the converging end, other things remaining equal, the volume fraction in the core decreases as R_a decreases. If there is a difference in the elasticity of various cells, a rigid cell will travel more slowly than more elastic cells, resulting in "bunching" of cells behind the rigid cell (Whitmore, 1967).

Theoretically, at a branch point in a capillary having about the same diameter as the cell, the branch with a faster stream gets most of the red cells because of the greater pressure gradient in that branch. Since, in addition, the net force is a vector pointing into the branch with a faster stream, both pressure and shear force tend to pull the red cell into the faster stream (Fung, 1973). This may explain in part the distribution of red cells among capillaries.

4.6 "STACKING" OF CELLS AND PLASMA MOTION BETWEEN CELLS

When the disc-diameter/tube-diameter ratio of biconcave discs is 0.9 or greater, the discs assume the "stacked" position as shown in Fig. 4.5 (Sutera and Hochmuth, 1968). When diameter ratios are 0.8 or less, cells may assume an "edge-on" flow position. Both cross-sectional shape and large diameter ratio are important factors in the normal stability of disclike particles in low Reynolds number tube flow, where plasma viscosity and flow is used to calculate the Reynolds number.

The relative velocity between plasma and cells establishes the criterion for the formation of circulation of plasma between red cells. No circulation results if the cell velocity is less than the average velocity of the plasma. When the cell velocity reaches the maximum velocity of the plasma, a stagnation region relative to the cell occurs near the center part of the capillary (Huang, 1971).

In the plasma trapped between two cells, an eddy current is theoretically formed because of the shear stresses acting on the plasma at the edge of the core. The eddy motions appear as in Fig. 4.5. This motion may contribute significantly to the transfer of solutes from the cell to the surrounding tissue. At least one unsuccessful attempt to observe plasma motion between cells in capillaries has been reported (Merrill and Wells, 1962). Prothero and Burton (1962) proposed a model for blood flow in capillaries in which the eddy currents in the plasma segments were important factors in the transfer of nutrients between the capillary wall and the erythrocyte. They used an analog experiment with water and an air segment to demonstrate the validity of this model. However, closer examination of the Prothero-Burton model indicated numerically that the analog experiments of the investigators were inappropriate. At least with oxygen and other dissolved gases, transfer through plasma is primarily diffusion controlled — the eddies take little part in the transfer (Aroesty and Gross, 1970).

When the Peclet number (Pe) or v_c/LD_i (where v_c is cell velocity, L is half the distance between cells, and D_i is diffusion coefficient for species). Brandt and Bugliarello (1965) and Bugliarello and Jackson (1964) have reported an approach to calculating the diffusion in plasma between cells using a "random walk" method. The entity to be diffused in the plasmatic gap — mass or heat — is simulated by mathematical "particles," which at each discrete time interval t^* execute two steps:

1. A convective step of length L_c, given by the distance traveled by the particle in time t^* under the action of the velocity field.

2. A diffusive step, random in direction but having a constant magnitude $L = \sqrt{2Dt^*}$.

The velocity field required as input to the convective step was developed for three-dimensional conditions and increasingly realistic erythrocyte shapes (Bugliarello and Hoskins, 1966).

The rate of oxygen transfer from cells can be calculated from a numerical solution of the convective diffusion equation by Bugliarello et al. (1969b). It was concluded that the motion in the plasmatic gaps contributed to oxygen transfer but that insufficient capillary length made this contribution unimportant.

The energy consumed in plasma eddy motion is partly responsible for an increase in pressure loss through the capillary. Cells closely stacked together theoretically reduce eddy current formation between the cells. Thus we must conclude that it takes no more energy to pass a densely packed train of cells through the capillary than a lightly packed one. In fact, if the energy loss in eddy motion is considered, there may even be less energy loss with more densely packed cells up to the point where they support one another and prevent distortion by the pressure gradient. This brings to mind the remark by Adams and Iampetro (1968) that the hemoconcentration initially accompanying high-altitude adaptation does not seem to impair capillary flow.

The pressure loss due to eddies in the plasma bolus between two red cells have been calculated for several idealized models (Lee and Fung, 1969; Bugliarello and Hsiao, 1970.) A solution for the pressure gradient due to eddies in the plasma bolus between two rigid flat surfaces as adapted from Lew and Fung appears in Fig. 4.8 as a plot of

$$\frac{\Delta P_c/\Delta x}{(\tau_{(R)}/4)} \quad \text{versus} \quad \frac{\Delta x}{r_c - \Delta r}$$

where $\Delta P_c/\Delta x$ = pressure gradient in bolus

Δx = distance between two red cells

This solution was derived originally for the case in which the cells filled the vessel. As described here, it is adapted to the case in which cells do not fill the tube, as in Fig. 4.5, where $r_c - \Delta r$ is the radius of the plasma bolus that varies as the cells deform under flow and $\tau_{(R)}$ is the shear stress at the point where the sheared plasma layer meets the plasma bolus (ie., when $R = r_c - \Delta r$).

The original solution presented by Lew and Fung plots is

$$\frac{\Delta P_c/\Delta x}{\mu_p \overline{V}/R_a} = \frac{\Delta P_c/\Delta x}{\tau_w/4}$$

It is the shear stress at the edge of the plasma bolus that governs its motion and pressure loss for a given geometry. The wall shear stress τ_w serves in the original solution because the cell fills the vessel and the edge of the bolus is at the wall. The model envisioned for the solution presented in Fig. 4.8 is a cylindrical plasma bolus bounded by two cells and surrounded by plasma in laminar flow (see Fig. 4.5). A curved cell surface at the ends of the bolus increases the pressure gradient when $\Delta x/r_c - \Delta r$ is greater than 1 (Bugliarello and Hsiao, 1970).

The total pressure gradient for the capillary is the sum of the pressure gradient (calculated without consideration of the bolus eddy flow) plus the pressure gradient calculated for the eddies, provided the eddy pressure gradient is small compared with the laminar flow pressure gradient. In the case of a relatively large eddy pressure gradient, a method of approximation would have to be employed to calculate the total pressure drop; that is, it would be necessary to calculate total pressure gradient, recheck $\tau_{(R)}$, recalculate $\Delta P_c/\Delta x$, recalculate new total pressure, and recheck $\tau_{(R)}$. When two successive $\tau_{(R)}$ values agree within reasonable limits, this can be related to the correct pressure gradient.

To estimate the order of magnitude of eddy pressure in a capillary consider Example 4.1. In this example the pressure gradient is calculated at the entrance section of a capillary without consideration of plasma eddies. The following information is given:

Blood flow rate	$= 3.7 \times 10^{-7}$ cm^3/sec
Plasma viscosity	$= 0.013$ P
Radius of capillary section	$= 5.26 \times 10^{-4}$ cm
Pressure gradient, (Calculated without eddy loss)	$= 0.198 \times 10^6$ dynes/cm^3
Radius of red cell, r_c	$= 4 \times 10^{-4}$ cm

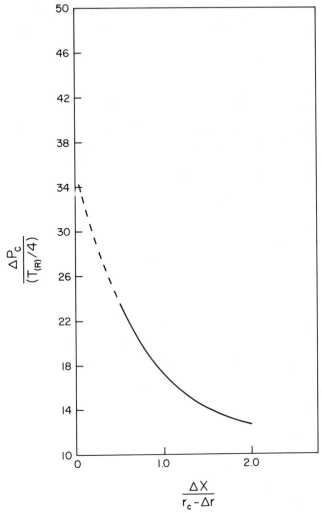

Fig. 4.8   Pressure loss due to eddies in plasma bolus as a function of distance between cells (adapted from Lew and Fung, 1969).

The value of Δr can be calculated from equation 4.10a; that is,

$$3.7 \times 10^{-7} = \frac{\pi(1.98 \times 10^{5})}{8(0.013)} \: [(5.26 \times 10^{-4})^{4} - (4 \times 10^{-4} - \Delta r)^{4}]$$

$$\Delta r = 4.8 \times 10^{-5} \text{ cm}$$
$$r_{c} - \Delta r = 3.52 \times 10^{-4} \text{ cm} = \text{plasma bolus radius}$$

Shear stress at edge of plasma bolus is

$$\tau_{(R)} = \frac{(1.98 \times 10^5)(3.52 \times 10^{-4})}{2} = 34.8 \text{ dynes/cm}^2$$

To determine length of plasma bolus Δx, assume a reservoir hematocrit of 45% or $\phi = 0.45$. Employing equation 4.16, we find the volume fraction of cells in the core:

$$\phi_c = \frac{0.45}{2}\left[\left(\frac{5.2 \times 10^{-4}}{3.52 \times 10^{-4}}\right)^2 + 1\right] = 0.7$$

The volume of the capillary core is $\pi(r_c - \Delta r)^2 \Delta L = 39.2 \times 10^{-10}$, and the volume of red cells in the core is $0.73 (39.2 \times 10^{-10}) = 28.6 \times 10^{-10} \text{ cm}^3$. Since the volume of a red cell V_0 is 84×10^{-12} there are $2860/84 = 34$ red cells in the capillary section at any time.

If red cell thickness is 1×10^{-4} cm, the plasma length between two isolated red cells is

$$\frac{0.01}{34} - 1 \times 10^{-4} = 1.95 \times 10^{-4} \text{ cm}$$

$$= \Delta x$$

and we have

$$\frac{\Delta x}{r_c - \Delta r} = \frac{1.95 \times 10^{-4}}{3.52 \times 10^{-4}} \cong 0.56$$

in Fig. 4.8

$$\frac{\Delta P_c}{\Delta x}\Bigg/\frac{\tau_{(R)}}{4} = 22 \qquad \text{for} \quad 0.56$$

Since $\tau_{(R)}/4 = 34.8/4 = 8.7$, $\Delta P_c/\Delta x = 8.7 \times 22 \cong 190$ dynes/cm^3.

This pressure gradient due to eddies in the plasma bolus is negligible compared with the laminar flow pressure gradient of 1.98×10^5 dynes/cm^3.

Since the values used in this example were of the order of those associated with the circulation, it appears that pressure gradients due to plasma eddies in capillaries are negligible. This is also confirmed by Fitz-Gerald (1972), who noted: "The maximum possible drop in the plasma boli, in fact, is very little more than the value expected for an equivalent length of cell-free plasma, under any circumstance of hematocrit and RBC distribution."

Owing to increasing the $(\Delta x/(r_c - \Delta r))$, pressure gradients associated with the plasma boli of groups of cells passing through the capillary are even lower than those of isolated cells (Bugliarello and Hsiao, 1970).

4.7   CELL MOVEMENT IN CAPILLARIES SMALLER THAN THE CELL

It has been frequently observed that red cells deform and flow through a capillary with radius smaller than that of the cell. Since most capillaries are smaller than red cells (Wiedeman, 1963; see Table 1.2), the cell flow described in this section theoretically predominates. The analysis of cell deformation described in the Appendix A4.1 applies here as in the case when the capillary radius was greater than cell radius.

When the cell is at rest in a capillary that has a radius smaller than its own, the primary force per unit of circumference of cell acting against or perpendicular to the wall is $(T \cos \theta)'$, which is given (see Section A4.1 and Fig. 4.9) by

$$(4.17) \quad (T \cos \theta)' = (r_c - R_a) E_c \left(\frac{R_a}{r_c}\right)^2$$

where T = horizontal force per unit circumference of cell in contact with capillary wall

θ = angle of cell contact with wall (see Fig. 4.7b)

E_c = elastic modulus of cell

In this case $r_c - R_a$ is the change from the unrestricted rest radius of the cell, since the radius of capillary is less than the radius of the cell by this amount. The wall is also exerting the same tension in the opposite direction on the cell, causing cell deformation and a decrease in the cell's projected radius from its unrestrained value r_c. When a pressure gradient P/L is applied across the cell, additional tension is exerted on the cell and further decrease in radius Δr occurs, as described by equation 4.8. For this case, however, with equation 4.8 the initial value of the vessel radius R_a is used for the red cell radius at rest r_c, since R_a is equal to the projected radius of the cell when there is no pressure gradient.

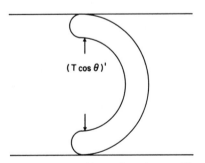

Fig. 4.9   Force pushing cell against capillary wall.

In the presence of a pressure gradient, Δr will be the distance between the edge of the cell and the vessel wall. The plasma between the cells can be considered as a first approximation to flow as a plug with the cells; the energy loss due to the eddy currents generated is assumed to be negligible.

The primary energy loss occurs in the sheared plasma layer between the plug and the wall. A straight-line velocity profile can be assumed between the edge of the plug or cells and the wall. Since plasma is a Newtonian fluid, equation 3.1 can be used to derive the relationship between pressure gradient and velocity:

$$(4.18) \quad \frac{P}{L} \frac{R_a}{2} = \mu_p \frac{v_c}{\Delta r}$$

and

$$(4.19) \quad Q = \pi (R_a - \Delta r)^2 v_c + 2\pi \left(R_a - \frac{\Delta r}{2} \right) \frac{v_c}{2} \Delta r$$

Equation 4.18 applies as long as a straight-line velocity profile exists. If Δr is more than 5% of R_a, equation 4.7 would be appropriate instead of 4.18; recalling that the initial or "rest" value of R_a is used to calculate Δr in equation 4.8. Thus the condition of a cell with a rest radius greater than the capillary radius is a special case of the more general model considered in Section 4.6.

There may be additional energy loss due to cell wall interactions and irregularities in wall and cell (e.g., in a bend of junction). There has been no quantitative experimental work along these lines with cells in vessels.

The principles applicable to flow in capillaries smaller than the cell are also described by lubrication theory (Fitz-Gerald, 1969).

Lubrication by a plasma film is a necessary feature of red cell movement in narrow capillaries. The plasma on a red cell constitutes a lubrication film between the cell and the endothelium. When some limiting film thickness is reached, the lubrication properties of the film disappear and cell seize-up occurs. When films are less than 500 Å thick, the lubricant behaves in a non-Newtonian manner, and there is an increase in resistance. The thin mucopolyssacharide coating on the endothelium probably forms such a limiting layer, and seize-up might be expected when this coating fills most of the lubrication region (Fitz-Gerald, 1969). The theory predicts, for example, that flow in a 7-μ capillary would cease at a pressure gradient of about 6 mm Hg/mm. Critical pressure gradients for smaller capillaries are much higher and seem to conflict with the results of Prothero and Burton (1962), who observed red cells passing through 5-μ millipore filter under a pressure of less than 4 cm H_2O. However, the red cell suspensions were very dilute. From equation 4.7, we can write

$$\text{film thickness} = \Delta r - r_c = \left[R_a{}^2 - \frac{4\mu_p L}{P} v_c \right]^{1/2}$$

which is in agreement with Fitz-Gerald's finding that film thickness varies with (velocity)$^{1/2}$.

Applying Fitz-Gerald's results to a capillary diameter 6×10^{-4} cm and a cell velocity of 0.012 cm/sec gives a lubrication film thickness of 10^{-5} cm; the leakback past the cell is 3.5% of the total flow. The mean resistance is about 5.5 times that for the whole blood Poiseuille flow (Gross and Aroesty, 1972). However, data obtained with 8-μ tubes do not agree with the predictions of lubrication theory (Barbee and Cokelet, 1972).

4.8   PLASMA FLOW IN PERICAPILLARY

It has been suggested that in certain organs a plasma annulus surrounds the capillary endothelium. The existence of a fluid pericapillary space was first demonstrated by Heimberger (1926). Gibson et al. (1956) observed a "pericapillary halo space" and noted that it appears in photomicrographs as a translucent space whose contour follows that of the capillary endothelia. Sapirstein (1958) proposed that the fluid annulus (supposed by Heimberger to contain lymph) actually contains plasma. Howe and Scheaffer (1966) mathematically analyzed Sapirstein's model; that is, a cylindrical endothelium tube of radius r_2 filled with a mixture of plasma and cells (see Fig. 4.10). The cells (radius r_1) move single file along the axis. The extra annulus of the plasma is between the endothelium and a larger concentric tube radius r_3. Hydrodynamic considerations lead to relationships between r_2 and r_3.

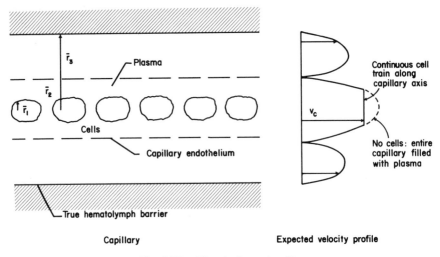

Fig. 4.10   Flow in the pericapillary.

For no annulus, Howe and Scheaffer showed that the ratio of capillary to large-vessel hematocrit is

$$(4.20) \quad \frac{Hc}{Hm} = 0.5 \left[1 + \left(\frac{\bar{r}_2}{\bar{r}_1} \right)^2 \right]$$

where Hc = the dynamic hematocrit of capillary
$\quad Hm$ = bulk hematocrit

(This is the same as equation 4.16 except that there is no allowance for cell deformation.)

Since r_2/r_1 lies between ∞ and 1, Howe and Scheaffer demonstrated that Hc/Hm is between 0.5 and 1. (It is indicated in Section 5.7 that Hc/Hm can be greater than 1 for this model.) However, they pointed out that Pappenheimer, who measured this ratio experimentally, found Hc/Hm as low as 0.35. Therefore, they concluded that the model without an annulus could not exist in this case. With plasma flow in the pericapillary, ratios of Hc/Hm as low as 0.27 could be obtained. Howe and Scheaffer further remarked that the ratio of Hc/Hm observed by Sapirstein could be explained on the basis of flow in a single capillary with or without the plasma annulus for the rat gut, heart, lungs, brain, and carcass. However, the ratios for the liver and kidney required the annulus model. With the annulus model it is possible to have ratios of Hc/Hm less than 1. Without an annulus, Howe and Scheaffer suggested that pressure—velocity data are in poor agreement. It is also noted that for high values of hematocrits, the peak velocity of the plasma in the annulus can exceed the cell velocity by a factor of 3 or more. Previously it was mentioned that cells lead the plasma in small vessels where the cells concentrate along the axial regions. However, a pericapillary annulus would allow the plasma flow to be less dependent on cell flow.

For a low ratio (such as in the liver), the peak velocity may be just a few percentage points of cell velocity. This suggests a possible mechanism for the observed disappearance and subsequent reappearance of labeled plasma in the microcirculation. Its prolonged absence may be caused by its slow movement along the annulus.

4.9   FLUID TRANSPORT THROUGH PORES IN CAPILLARY WALL

Since the transfer of water across capillary walls influences flow in the microcirculation, it is appropriate to consider this phenomenon briefly. Passage through pores in the capillary wall is the favored mechanism for the transport of water across the wall. The capillary pore, which is thought to be at the junction of the endothelial cells making up the wall, has a radius of about 4×10^{-7} cm.

The thickness of capillary wall is 0.5×10^{-4} cm (Landis and Pappenheimer, 1963). The volume flow of solution across the capillary wall (filtration flow) is given by

(4.21) $Q_v = [(P - P^1) - (P_o - P_o')] L_p$

where P = hydrostatic pressure in capillary
             P^1 = hydrostatic pressure tissue
             P_o, P_o' = osmotic pressure in capillary and tissue, respectively
             L_p = filtration coefficient (see below)

The water flow is in the opposite direction to the osmotic pressure gradient (see Fig. 4.11); however, water flow will always be in the direction of its partial pressure gradient or its chemical potential gradient. The filtration coefficient can be represented as

$$L_p = \frac{\pi}{t_p \, 8 \, \mu} R_p^{\,4}$$

where μ = viscosity of water
        t_p = pore length
        R_p = radius of pore

The filtration coefficient for a porous membrane in the forearm capillary 5×10^{-5} cm thick is 5.7×10^{-3} ml/min/(mm Hg)/(100 g of tissue), (Landis and Gibbon, 1933; Wiener and Silberberg, 1968).

Using an osmotic pressure of 7.6 mm Hg and a filtration coefficient of $0.0816 \ \mu^3/(\mu^2)$(sec)(mm Hg), pressures in the frog mesentery capillaries are calculated to be about 12 mm Hg at the arteriolar end and 7 mm Hg at the venous end (Intaglietta and Zweifach, 1966). The filtration rate per unit area is in the order of $0.05 \ \mu^3/(\mu^2)$(sec)(mm Hg) with vessel diameter between $22 \ \mu$ at the arteriolar end and $17 \ \mu$ at the venous end. In the rat omentum, filtration coefficients $0.01 \ \mu^3/(\mu^2)$(sec)(mm Hg) were calculated. Of the capillaries tested, 70 to 80% lost fluid because their blood hydraulic pressure was higher than colloidal osmotic pressure.

Equation 4.21, known as Starling's hypothesis, applies to ideal membranes that do not allow solute (in this case protein) to "leak." However, the capillary wall is not an ideal membrane, and solute (e.g., small amounts of albumin) passes through. Under these circumstances the volume flow rate of solution and the flow of solute are related to the osmotic pressure and hydrostatic pressure by principles of nonequilibrium thermodynamics (e.g., Katchalsky and Curran, 1965).

(4.22) $Q_v = \dfrac{\pi}{8\mu_p L} R_p^{\,4} \left[(P_1 - P') - \sigma(P_o - P_o')\right]$

where σ is the reflection coefficient of protein in plasma.

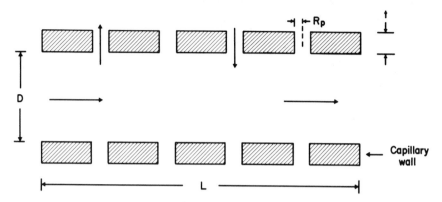

Fig. 4.11 Simplified schematic diagram of porous capillary wall showing outflow of water due to hydrostatic pressure and absorption due to osmotic pressure.

The flow rate of solute across the wall is

(4.23) $Q_D = C_S(1 - \sigma)Q_v + w(P_o - P_o')$

where C_s = concentration of solute
w = solute mobility or permeability coefficient

Thorough discussions of restricted and free diffusion of molecules across capillary walls are given by Landis and Pappenheimer (1963) and Dick (1966).

By assuming a set of pore dimensions suggested by electron microscope studies, the pore model of Pappenheimer et al. (1951) has been modified by Lifson (1970) and Tosteson (1970) to include irreversible thermodynamic treatments of parallel pore, cell pathway and constricted pore effects (Perl, 1971). The Pappenheimer data can be separated into permeability w and reflection coefficient σ, which show good agreement with more recent experimental data; see Table 4.6.

The osmotic pressure due to proteins in plasma is called the oncotic pressure. Since the pH of plasma is on the alkaline side of the isoelectric point of most proteins, these exist as large multivalent anions. The capillary wall restricts the protein while allowing free diffusion of most other smaller ions. The distribution of smaller ions is not equal, however, either because of the Donnan effect or because the electrochemical potential on both sides of the wall must be equal. Accounting for the small ion difference across the capillary wall caused by the Donnan equilibrium effect, the osmotic pressure difference across the wall is written (Scatchard et al., 1946)

(4.24) $\Delta P_o = RT \left((Pr) + \dfrac{Z^2 (Pr)^2}{4Ms} \right)$

Table 4.6 Reflection σ and Permeability W Coefficients[a]

Solute	σ^b	σ^c	W^d (cm/sec $\times 10^5$)	W^e (cm/sec $\times 10^5$)	W^f (cm/sec $\times 10^5$)
Nacl	0.16	–	5.0	7.4	3.8
Urea	0.21	0.10	4.8	6.1	3.1
Glucose	0.22	–	2.0	2.7	1.0
Sucrose	0.29	0.30	1.5	1.8	0.8
Raffinose	0.30	0.38	1.2	1.1	–
Imulin	0.54	0.69	0.27	0.27	0.27

[a]From Perl (1971).
[b]Calculated results from Pappenheimer et al (1951).
[c]Experimental results of Vargas and Johnson (1964).
[d]Calculated results from Pappenheimer (1951).
[e]Experimental permeability coefficients from Trap-Jensen and Lassen (1970).
[f]Experimental permeability coefficients from Alvarez and Yudilevich (1969).

where $\quad R =$ gas constant $= 62.4\ (mmHg)(L)/^\circ K\ (mole)$

$\quad T =$ absolute temperature

$\quad Pr =$ protein concentration inside capillary (moles/l)

$\quad Z =$ net charge on protein

$\quad Ms =$ moles of salt outside capillary

$Z^2 (Pr)^2 / 4Ms =$ difference in salt concentration across wall

The difference in salt concentration between inside and outside the capillaries is about 6.2×10^{-4} moles/L. The salt concentration outside the capillary is about 0.15 mole/L. This relatively small difference in salt concentration accounts for about half the osmotic pressure difference across the capillary wall. For plasma $Z = 26.5$, $Pr = 7.31 \times 10^{-4}$ mole/L, and $Ms = 0.15$ mole/L. Binding of Cl^- and protein interaction cause deviations from equation 4.24.

Net charge is a function of pH, which is relatively constant, as is the salt concentration outside in tissue. The change in osmotic pressure difference $d(\Delta P_o)$ with change in plasma protein molar concentration Pr is found by differentiating equation 4.24:

$$(4.25) \qquad d(\Delta P_o) = RT \left(dPr + \frac{Z^2}{4Ms} (2) (Pr) d(Pr) \right) = RT [2.7\ d(Pr)]$$

Since water transfers across the capillary wall, the protein concentration must vary along the capillary, causing a change in the osmotic pressure difference along the capillary (see Example 4.2). The transmural pressure will be influenced, and consequently capillary radius and flow through the capillary pore will be affected.

Gordon (1969) has cited the results of glucose clearance tests, as an example of the influence of osmotic effects on transcapillary flow. Glucose affects osmotic pressure in capillaries, leading to the withdrawal of sufficient water from tissues to cause a 2% hemodilution, consequently reducing blood viscosity. Colloid osmotic pressure is related to mean blood pressure but is independent of hematocrit. It varies considerably within a species (Intaglietta and Zweifach, 1971).

The internal pressure at any point in the capillary is affected by the mechanical properties of the wall and the cells and by the plasma viscosity. These properties also influence the absorption or expulsion of fluid from the capillary by hydrostatic—osmotic pressure, which is determined in part by energy loss due to flow in the capillary.

Measurements of transcapillary fluid exchange in single capillaries reveal that the venous capillary has a higher filtration than does the arterial segment (Zweifach and Intaglietta, 1968). Coupled with the observation that the venous capillary is larger, this finding suggests that the midpoint of capillary fluid exchange in the context of the classical Starling hypothesis is well into the venous side of the capillary (Johnson, 1972).

Wiederhielm (1968) carried out computer analysis of fluid balance in capillary flow. He considered four fluid fluxes into and out of the interstitial space: filtration, reabsorption, plasma leakage through large pore system, and removal of tissue fluid by lymphatic substances. The program also took into account changes in tissue fluid protein concentration as determined by differences in the protein fluxes into the interstitial space through the large pore system in a capillary, as well as protein removal by the lymphatics. He did not consider the effect of red cell or vessel wall elasticity characteristics on capillary hydrostatic pressure, yet he found qualitative agreement with clinical data.

If the corpuscles just fit the capillary (see Section 5.9), as is common, the cell and capillary walls are in close contact, and water probably moves across both walls direct from the interstitial fluid to the red cell interior without passing through the plasma (Hansen, 1961).

Such a mechanism could explain the daily transfer of about 36 L of water from the interstitial fluid to the blood. In addition, it is independent of the osmotic pressure of the plasma proteins that, following the conventional Starling-Landis theory, govern transcapillary water shifts (Dick, 1966). Hansen's proposal, according to Dick, accounts for the superiority of a transfusion of whole blood over that of plasma in the relief of edema. If red cells are for any reason reduced in size (e.g., as in microcytic anemia), they are not in direct contact with the capillary wall, and the water they take up comes largely from the plasma and not from the interstitial fluid. The edema that is characteristic of microcytic anemia is thus accounted for. However, direct demonstration of water transfer from tissue fluid to red cell is still lacking.

4.10   TRANSPORT OF HEMOGLOBIN IN CELLS VERSUS HEMOGLOBIN IN SOLUTION

Which method provides the more efficient transport of hemoglobin — hemoglobin packaged in cells or hemoglobin free in plasma?

A hemoglobin solution having the same oxygen-carrying capacity as a suspension of red cells has a lower viscosity than the red cell suspension (Schmidt-Nielson and Taylor, 1968; Cokelet and Meiselman, 1968). Canine blood ($\phi = 0.45$, hemoglobin 14.8 g/100 ml) has a viscosity of 0.047 P, whereas the hemoglobin from the cells has a viscosity of 0.033 P. The plasma viscosity is 0.0175 P (Schmidt-Nielson and Taylor, 1968).

The flow of a hemoglobin solution in plasma passing through a 10-μ capillary is calculated to be the same as a suspension of red cells having the same oxygen-carrying capacity. However, the diameters of the major resistance vessels are in the order of 50 to 100 μ. The flow rate of the hemoglobin solution in a

100-μ tube is 30% greater than if the same hemoglobin were contained in cells; the flow of hemoglobin in a 70-μ tube is 13% greater than the red cell suspension. The equations for calculations in these tubes are in Chapter 3.

Thus we can conclude that transport of hemoglobin in solution is more efficient than transport in cells, (see p. 54).

Example 4.1

(*a*) Determine the vessel shape and flow rate through a capillary given the following information:

Osmotic pressure difference across wall P_o	= 25 mm Hg
	= 0.33 x 10^5 dynes/cm^2
Tissue hydrostatic pressure	= 0
Entrance pressure P_1	= 32 mm Hg
	= 0.426 x 10^5 dynes/cm^2
Exit pressure P_{10}	= 0.200 x 10^5 dynes/cm^2
Length L	= 0.1 cm
ΔL	= 0.01 cm
Wall elastic modulus E_w	= 10^6 dynes/cm^2
Wall Poisson ratio	= 0.25
Wall thickness "at rest" T_0	= 1 x 10^{-4}
Vessel radius "at rest" R_0	= 5 x 10^{-4} cm
Plasma viscosity μ_p	= 0.013 P
Radius of cell "at rest" r_c	= 4 x 10^{-4} cm
Elastic modulus of cell E_c	= 5 x 10^7 dynes/cm^2
Radius of thick region of cell a	= 1 x 10^{-4} cm
Poisson ratio of red cell ν_c	= 0.3
Volume of red cell V_0	= 84 x 10^{-12} cm^3

Solution

Employ procedure outlined in Section 4.4, considering the capillary to be divided into 10 segments as in Fig. 4.2. Now perform the following calculations:

$$\frac{\Delta P_1}{\Delta L} = \frac{0.426 \times 10^5 - 0.200 \times 10^5}{0.1} = 0.226 \times 10^6 \text{ dynes/cm}^3$$

or $\Delta P_1 = 0.226 \times 10^6 \times 10^{-2} = 0.226 \times 10^4$ dynes/cm^2
$P_2 = 0.426 \times 10 \times 0.226 \times 10^4 = 0.948 \times 10^5$ dynes/cm^2
$P_1 = 0.426 \times 10^5$ dynes/cm^2
$P_t = 0.426 \times 10^5 - 0.333 \times 10^5 = 0.086 \times 10^4$ dynes/cm^2

From equation 4.5 we can write

$$\frac{(R_a)_1}{5 \times 10^{-4}} = \frac{(8.6 \times 10^2)(5 \times 10^{-4})}{10^6 \times 10^{-4}} \left(\frac{R_{a_1}}{5 \times 10^{-4}}\right)^{0.3} + 1$$

Having found R_{a_1}, find Q using equation 4.10:

$$Q = \frac{\pi}{8(0.013)} (0.226 \times 10^6) [R_{a_1}{}^4 - (4 \times 10^{-4} - \Delta r)^4]$$

Next use equation 4.8 to determine Δr

$$\Delta r = \frac{3(84 \times 10^{-12})(4 \times 10^{-4})^2}{(1 \times 10^{-4})^2} \left[\frac{0.226 \times 10^6}{(4 \times 10^{-4} - \Delta r)^5 (5 \times 10^7)(1 - 0.3)^2}\right]^{1/3}$$
$$\cos\left[\frac{1}{2} \left\{\frac{0.226 \times 10^6}{5 \times 10^7} (4 \times 10^{-4} - \Delta r)[24 (1 - 0.3)]\right\}^{1/3}\right]$$

To find $(R_a)_2$, and Q knowing P_2, solve equations 4.8 and 4.10 simultaneously for Δr and $(\Delta P/\Delta L)_2$. This must be done with a computer. When $(\Delta P/\Delta L)_2$ has been determined, $(\Delta P)_2$ is found from $(\Delta P/\Delta L)_2 \Delta L = \Delta P_2$. Now $P_3 = P_2 + \Delta P_2$. Similarly $(R_a)_3$ is found $(\Delta P/\Delta L)_3$ and P_3. When we know ΔP_1 through ΔP_{10}, the sum of these is compared with $P_1 - P_{10}$. If they agree, Q is correct and Ra versus L is correct. If they do not agree, another trial is made by adjusting $\Delta P/\Delta L$. The computer program for this calculation is in Section A4.3, Fig. A4.5. The calculated shape of the capillary appears in Fig. 4.2.

To use the computer program for making the calculation just described, initial estimates of $(\Delta P/\Delta L)$, (R_a), and Δr must be supplied as indicated in the read statement of the program. The initial $(\Delta P/\Delta L)$, can be estimated as shown in the first step of the solution; (R_a), can be guesstimated as 6×10^{-4} cm and Δr as 2×10^{-4} cm. These are adjusted in the program to their correct values, but the closer the estimates, the less the computer time required.

The flow rate in this example is 3.7×10^{-7} cm^3/sec. Final pressure gradient for the first section is $(\Delta P_1/\Delta L) = 0.198 \times 10^6$ dynes/cm^3. The radius as a function of distance along the capillary is noted in Table 4.2, along with the pressure drop in each section. The pressure drop is not linear along the capillary length. In this case there is about a 10% difference in radius between entrance and exit.

Estimation of Average Viscosity in a Capillary

Using Poiseuille's equation to calculate apparent viscosity along the capillary, we find that the apparent viscosities at the entrance and exit sections are 0.0158 and 0.033 P, respectively. Thus the average viscosity along the capillary is

0.025 P, which is in agreement with the experimental value of Prothero and Burton (1962) — namely, 0.02 P, found in 5 to 10 μ glass capillary tubes; see Section 4.6.

(b) Solve for the pressure drop in a capillary, for the conditions noted in Example 4.1a using the method of Sutera et al. (1970); see equation 4.11. To use this method the cell velocity must be known.

The flow rate determined in Example 4.1a is 3.7×10^{-7} cm^3/sec. From this it is possible to calculate first the gap between cell and wall, using equation 4.10, and then red cell velocity, using equation 4.7.

The mean velocity $\overline{V}$ is $(3.7 \times 10^{-7})/(25 \times 10^{-8}) = 0.47$ cm/sec, and

$$\frac{\mu_p \overline{V}}{E_c D_t} = \frac{(0.013)(0.47)}{(5 \times 10^7)(10^{-3})} = 1.222 \times 10^{-7}$$

$$\frac{D_c}{D_t} = \frac{8 \times 10^{-4}}{1 \times 10^{-3}} = 0.8$$

From Fig. 4.7 we can write

$$\frac{\Delta P^*}{\mu_p \cdot \overline{V}/D_t} \cong 10$$

If a pressure gradient of 2.26×10^5 dynes/cm^3 is assumed as a first approximation the $r_c - \Delta r$ can be calculated from equation 4.10; that is, we can put

$$3.7 \times 10^{-7} = \frac{(2.26 \times 10^5)\pi}{8(0.013)} [5 \times 10^{-4})^4 - (r_c - \Delta r)^4]$$

$$(r_c - \Delta r) = 3.35 \times 10^{-4} \text{ cm}$$

From equation 4.10, v_c is found to be 0.645 cm/sec. Employing equation 4.11 and assuming a hematocrit of 45%, we write

$$\Delta P_{cell} = (0.45)(0.47)\frac{(\pi)(10^{-3})^2}{4} \frac{(0.1)}{(0.645)} \left(\frac{1}{84} \times 10^{-12}\right) (10)(1.22 \times 10^{-7})$$

$$(5 \times 10^7)$$

$$\Delta P_{cell} = 2.4 \times 10^3 \text{ dynes/cm}^2$$

$$\Delta P_{Pois} = 32 \frac{(1.3 \times 10^{-2})(0.4^7)(10^{-1})}{(10^{-3})(10^{-3})} = 19.5 \times 10^3$$

$$\Delta P_{cells} + \Delta P_{Pois} = 2.19 \times 10^4 \text{ dynes/cm}^2$$

or

overall pressure gradient $= 2.19 \times 10^5$ dynes/cm^3

This is in close agreement with the 2.26×10^5 assumed in the calculation of $r_c - \Delta r$ and computed from Example 4.1a.

Example 4.2

What effect will a 1.5% decrease in plasma protein have on the transmural pressure at the entrance to the capillary?

Given

Hydrostatic pressure at capillary entrance = 32 mm Hg
Osmotic pressure acting across capillary
wall to move water into capillary   = 28 mm Hg

Solution

Use equation 4.25, $d(P_r) = 1 \times 10^{-5+}$ moles/L. Thus we have

$$d(\Delta P) = 62.4(310)\,(2.7)\,(-1 \times 10^{-5}) = -0.55 \text{ mm Hg}$$

Initial transmural pressure is $32 - 28 = 4$ mm Hg.

After protein change, transmural pressure is $32 - 27.45 = 4.5$ mm Hg; or about 10% change in transmural pressure is caused by a 1.5% change in protein concentration.

APPENDIX   DERIVATIONS OF CELL FLEXIBILITY AND CAPILLARY FLOW EQUATIONS

A4.1   Velocity of Red Cell in a Capillary

The velocity of the cell in a capillary is the same as the velocity at the streamline at the edge of the cell, which is at a distance $r_c - \Delta r$ from the center (r_c = cell radius at rest; Δr = change in cell radius due to distortion); see Fig. 4.4.

The point velocity of the plasma is found from

$$(A4.1) \qquad \frac{P}{2L} \int_{r_c - \Delta r}^{Ra} R\, dR = \mu_p \int_{v}^{0} -\, dv$$

$$v_P = \frac{P}{4\mu L}\, [Ra^2 - (r_c - \Delta r)^2]$$

where v_P is the velocity of plasma at edge of the red cell.

If plasma should possess a yield stress, equation A4.1 becomes

$$\text{(A4.2)} \quad v_P = \frac{P}{4\mu_P L} (R^2 - (r_c - \Delta r)^2) + \frac{4}{3\mu_p} \left[\frac{PC}{2L}\right]^{1/3}$$

$$[R^{3/2} - (r_c - \Delta r)^{3/2}] + \frac{C}{\mu_P} [R - (r_c - \Delta r)]$$

Cell distortion in flow.   Cell distortion due to pressure gradient across a cell can be determined by considering the forces acting on a cell in a capillary. The cell is idealized to appear in cross section as in Fig. 4.3 (i.e., a torus encircling a disc).

When a cell flow exists in a capillary, as in Fig. A4.1, a net drag force S acts on the torus and a pressure load P/L (t_c) acts in the opposite direction on the central portions of the cell. In reference to Fig. A4.1, T is the force per unit of a circumference exerted on torus by the central membrane of the cell, a is the radius of the torus, r_c is the cell radius at rest, and S is the drag force.

Forces acting on the torus in Fig. A4.1 can be resolved into an equivalent force system of a horizontal component and a moment for S and a horizontal and vertical component for T (see Fig. A4.2). If the velocity of the cell is constant, there can be no net force acting on the cell, and $S = T \sin \theta$. The moment Sa acts uniformly all around the torus and is therefore self-equilibrating (see Fig. A4.3). It is assumed that the twisting action of the distributed moment does not grossly deform the membrane. The distributed force $T \cos \theta$ is the force of primary concern, since it causes a radial contraction of the torus (see Fig. A4.4). The circumferential stress in the torus is approximately

$$\text{(A4.3)} \quad S_c = \frac{T r_c \cos \theta}{\pi a^2}$$

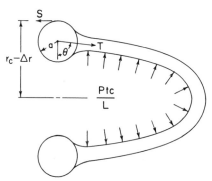

Fig. A4.1   Forces acting on an idealized cell in capillary flow.

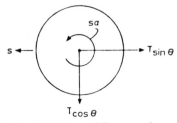

Fig. A4.2   Resolution of Forces acting on circular edge of torus.

and the circumferential strain is

$$(A4.4) \quad \frac{\Delta r}{r_c} = \frac{T r_c \cos \theta}{\pi E_c a^2}$$

or

$$(A4.5) \quad \Delta r = \frac{T \cos \theta}{\pi E_c} \left(\frac{r_c}{a}\right)^2$$

It is now necessary to relate T and θ to the geometric and material properties and the applied loading $Pt_c L$ across the cell.

Consider the central portion of the cell. It has previously been observed that red cells deform in the shape of a paraboloid. Thus we have

$$(A4.6) \quad w = \frac{P}{L} t_c \frac{r^2}{4T} + \text{constant}$$

where w = lateral displacement of membrane

r = radial distance measured from axis of symmetry

Differentiating equation A4.6 gives

$$(A4.7) \quad \left(\frac{dw}{dr}\right)_{r=(r_c - \Delta r)} = \frac{Pt_c(r_c - \Delta r)}{2LT} = \tan \theta$$

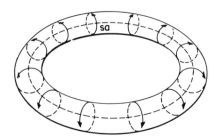

Fig. A4.3   Moment acting on torus edge of cell is self equilibrating.

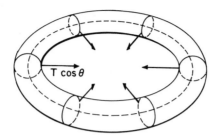

Fig. A4.4   The force component $T \cos \theta$ causes a contraction of the edge.

Assuming that $\tan \theta$ can be replaced by θ – for $\theta \leq 30°$ the error is 10% – we can write

(A4.8) $\theta = \dfrac{Pt_c(r_c - \Delta r)}{2LT}$

Now T is related to the applied pressure by noting that an originally flat membrane loaded by a uniform pressure will deflect into a spherical segment and that (Den Hartog, 1952):

(A4.9) $T = t_c \left[\dfrac{E_c(r_c - \Delta r)^2 \ (P/L)^2}{24(1 - \nu_c)} \right]^{1/3}$

If the paraboloid is shallow, equation A4.9 is accurate, for under these conditions the distinction between a paraboloid and a spherical segment can be ignored. When the membrane deflection is large, a nonlinear analysis is required and equation A4.9 gives only an approximation. Assuming that the approximation is adequate for these purposes and substituting equations A4.9 and A4.8 into A4.5, we obtain

(A4.10) $\Delta r = \dfrac{r_c^2 t_c [(r_c - \Delta r)^2]^{1/3}}{\pi [24(1 - \nu_c)^{1/3}] a^2} \left(\dfrac{P}{LE_c} \right)^{2/3}$

$$\left\{ \cos \left[\dfrac{1}{2} \left\{ \dfrac{P}{E_c L} (r_c - \Delta r) \ [24(1 - \nu_c)] \right\}^{1/3} \right] \right\}$$

In addition, the thickness t_c is a function of Δr. This relationship can be determined by assuming that the volume of the cell V_o is constant and that

(A4.11) $V_o = A t_c$

where A is the surface area of one side of the cell.

It is possible to determine A from the trace of the distorted cells as described by equation A4.6. The constant in equation A4.6 is found by assigning $w = 0$ at

$r = r_c - \Delta r$. Substituting these values in equation A4.6, we learn that the constant is

$$-\frac{P}{L}(r_c - \Delta r)^2 \bigg/ \left[\frac{E_c(r_c - \Delta r)^2 (P/L)^2}{24(1 - \nu_c)} \right]^{1/3}$$

The displacement w as function of the distance from the center r is found from equation A4.6. Note that the values of w will appear to be negative. This is merely because the direction of r was chosen in a manner that makes r decrease as w increases. The surface area of one side of the cell can now be found from a consideration of the surface of revolution generated by the trace of the paraboloid cell. Thus we have

$$(A4.12) \quad A = \int_0^{w_{max}} 2\pi r \, dw = \frac{P}{L} t_c \int_0^{r_c - \Delta r} \pi r \left(\frac{r}{T} \right) dr$$

$$A = \frac{\pi P (r_c - \Delta r)^3}{3L} \left[\frac{24(1 - \nu_c)}{E_c (P/L)^2 (r_c - \Delta r)} \right]^{1/3}$$

Substituting this for A in equation A4.11, solving for T_c, and substituting for T_c in equation A4.10, we find equation (4.8), or

$$\Delta r = 3V_0 r_c^2 \left[\frac{t_c}{(r_c - \Delta r)^5 E_c 24(1 - \nu_c)^2} \right]^{1/2}$$

$$\cos \frac{1}{2} \left[\frac{P}{E_c L}(r_c - \Delta r)(24(1 - \nu_c)) \right]^{1/3}$$

A4.2   Volume Fraction of Cells Flowing in Single File along Capillary as Function of Reservour Concentration

$$\frac{\phi(Q)}{Q_c} = \phi_c = \frac{\phi(\pi P/8\mu_p L)[R_a^4 - (r_c - \Delta r)^4]}{\pi P/4\mu_p L [R_a^2 - (r_c - \Delta r)^2] (r_c - \Delta r)^2}$$

$$Q_c = \frac{\phi}{2} \left[\frac{R_a^2 + (r_c - \Delta r)^2}{(r_c - \Delta r)^2} \right] = \frac{\phi}{2} \left[\frac{R_a^2}{(r_c - \Delta r)^2} + 1 \right]$$

where Δr is given by equation 4.8.

A4.3   Computer Program Used for Chapter 4

```
C        DR', CHARM DISTENSIBLE TUBE PRESSURE/FLOW/RADIUS PROGRAM
       1 READ (1,1000) RO,XNU,EW,TO,VC,RC,A,EC,XC,XMU,XK1,XK2,XK3,XK4,XK5,
        1XK6,XK7
    1000 FORMAT (8E10,4)
      10 DO 500 ICYCLE=1,20
         P1=XK1
         P10=XK3
         DO 400 ISTEP=1,10
         PT=P1-XK2
         IF (PT) 15,15,20
      15 R=RLAST
         GO TO 40
      20 RLAST=XK4
         DO 35 J=1,10
         J=J
         R=RO*(((PT*RO)/(EW*TO)*(RLAST/RO)**(XNU)+1,)
         IF (ABS((R-RLAST)/RLAST)-,05) 40,40,35
      35 RLAST=R
C
      40 RLAST=R
         IF (ISTEP-1) 45,45,50
      45 DRLAST=XK6
         DO 55 K=1,20
         K=K
         DR=((3,*VC*RC**2)/(3,14157*A**2))
         DR=DR*(XK5/((RC-DRLAST)**5*EC*24,*(1,-XC)**2))**,33333
         DR=DR*COS(,5*((XK5/EC)*(RC-DRLAST)*(24,*(1,-XC)))**,33333)
         IF (RC-DR) 46,54,54
      46 WRITE (3,1400) RC,DR,DRLAST
    1400 FORMAT (15X,52HRC IS LESS THAN DR-CONVERGENCE HAS BEEN FORCED    RC
        1=,E10,4,3X,3HDR=E10,4,3X,7HDRLAST=,E10,4)
         DR=DRLAST
         GO TO 60
      54 IF (ABS((DR-DRLAST)/DRLAST)-,05) 60,60,55
      55 DRLAST=DR
C
      60 Q=(3,14157*XK5/(8,*XMU))*(R**2+   (RC-DR)**2)*(R**2-(RC-DR)**2)
         CALL FORDTE (A1,A2)
         WRITE (3,1100) A1,A2,ICYCLE,XK1,XK3,XK5,Q
    1100 FORMAT (10H1DR, CHARM,75X,2A4//4X,5HCYCLE,I3,3X,3HP1=,E10,4,3X,
        14HP10=,E10,4,3X,4HP/L=,E10,4,3X,2HQ=E10,4)
         WRITE (3,1500) XNU,EW,TO,VC,RC,A,EC,XC
    1500 FORMAT ( /5H XNU=,E10,4,4H EW=,E10,4,4H XC=,E10,4,4H VC=,E10,4,
        14H RC=,E10,4,3H A=,E10,4,4H EC=,E10,4,4H XC=,E10,4)
         WRITE (3,1600)
    1600 FORMAT                                    (/12X,4HSTEP,6X,2HPT,
        29X,4HP(I),6X,7HDELTA P,7X,1HR,9X,7HDELTA R,4X,6HR ITER,3X,
        38HP/L ITER/)
C
         DPDL=XK5
      70 DP=XK7*DPDL
         WRITE (3,1200) ISTEP,PT,P1,DP,R,DR,J,K
    1200 FORMAT (14X,I2,5E12,4,I7,I11)
         P1=P1-DP
         GO TO 400
C
      50 DRLAST=XK6
         DO 75 K=1,20
         
         DPDL=(Q*8,*XMU)/(3,14157*(R**4-(RC-DRLAST)**4))
         DR=((3,*VC*RC**2)/(3,14157*A**2))
         DR=DR*(DPDL/((RC-DRLAST)**5*EC*24,*(1,-XC)**2))**,33333
         DR=DR*COS(,5*((DPDL/EC)*(RC-DRLAST)*(24,*(1,-XC)))**,33333)
         IF (RC-DR) 76,74,74
```

```
   76 WRITE (3,1400) RC,DR,DRLAST
      DR=DRLAST
      GO TO 70
   74 IF (ABS((DR=DRLAST)/DRLAST)=.C1) 70,70,75
   75 DRLAST=DP
      GO TO 70
C
  600 CONTINUE
      PLAST=P1+LP
      IF (ABS((XK3=PLAST)/PLAST)=.01) 8C,80,85
   80 GO TO 1
   85 IF (XK3=PLAST) 90,90,95
   90 XK5=XK5+.03*XK5
      GO TO 500
   95 XK5=XK5=.02*XK5
  500 CONTINUE
      WRITE (3,1300)
 1300 FORMAT (//////34H HAS NOT CONVERGED AFTER 20 CYCLES)
      GO TO 1
      END
```

Fig. A4.5   *Read Statement Definitions:* RO = R_0; XNV = v; EW = E_w; TO = T_0; VC = $\overline{V}_C$; RC = r_C; A = a; EC = E_C; XC = v_C; XMU = μ_p; XK1 = P_1; XK2 = ΔP_0 osmotic pressure difference; XK3 = P_{10}; XK4 = estimate of initial value of R_a in first section; XK5 = estimate of initial value of ($\Delta P/\Delta L$); XK6 = estimate of Δr in first section; XK7 = ΔL. (See Example 4.1).

Blood Viscosity in Heat and Mass Transfer

Chapter 5

HEAT AND MASS TRANSFER are governed by the same operational principles as fluid flow, that is,

$$\text{rate of transfer} = \frac{\text{driving force}}{\text{resistance}}$$

In *ex vivo* systems the influence of viscosity on mass and heat transfer has been studied extensively with various fluids and systems. However, there have been very few studies of heat transfer and almost none of mass transfer with respect to the influence of plasma and blood viscosity. In this section the general concepts used in mass and heat transfer calculations are applied to blood and plasma in the circulation to suggest an approach.

5.1 BLOOD VISCOSITY IN HEAT TRANSFER

Viscosity influences heat transfer through its effect on fluid resistance to heat transfer and indirectly through its effect on flow rate. Several resistances are encountered in the transfer of heat to or from blood flowing in a vessel: resistance of the blood of the vessel wall with surrounding tissue and resistance of the outside environment (see Figs. 5.1 and 5.2).

It has been found that when yield stress effects are negligible, blood viscosity per se has little direct effect on heat transfer resistance (Mitvalsky, 1965; Charm

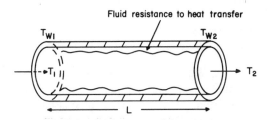

Fig. 5.1   Resistances to heat transfer.

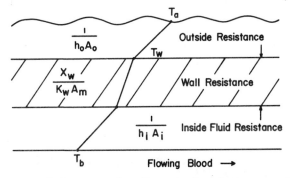

Fig. 5.2   Detailed representation of heat transfer resistance at a wall section.

171

et al., 1968b). The resistance R_f to heat transfer associated with a fluid flowing inside a cylindrical tube or vessel is

(5.1) $R_f = \dfrac{1}{h_i A_i}$

where R_f = fluid resistance to heat transfer
h_i = heat transfer coefficient associated with fluid
A_i = lateral surface area inside tube wetted by fluid

The heat transfer coefficient for blood can be evaluated from the Sieder-Tate equation (Sieder-Tate, 1936):

(5.2) $\dfrac{h_i D}{k} = 1.75 \left(\dfrac{WC_P}{kL}\right)^{1/3} \left(\dfrac{\mu_w}{K_B{}^2}\right)^{0.14}$ for $\dfrac{WC}{kL} > 6;$

for $\dfrac{WC}{kL} < 6$, use Fig. 5.3.

where

W = mass flow rate of blood through vessel or tube
k = thermal conductivity of blood
L = length of vessel or tube
C_p = specific heat of blood
h_i = heat transfer coefficient for blood flowing inside a vessel or tube
D = diameter of vessel
μ_w = apparent viscosity at wall
$K_B{}^2$ = viscosity of blood at bulk average temperature

The viscosity term $(\mu_w/K_B{}^2)^{0.14}$ is required to correct for deviations from a parabolic velocity profile when caused either by temperature variations or cell distributions along the radius. When marginal plasma layer or cell distribution across the radius exists, μ_w is the plasma viscosity at the wall temperature and $K_B{}^2$ is the suspension apparent viscosity at the bulk average temperature. When tube diameters are greater than 155 μ and hematocrits greater than 40, μ_w is the apparent viscosity of blood at the temperature of the wall.

Mitvalsky (1965) determined the heat transfer coefficients for blood flowing through a tube 1 cm in diameter and an annulus 0.185 cm in diameter for the case where WC/KL is greater than 6. Good agreement is found between his results and equation 5.2. Figure 5.3 was determined using diameters 0.0162 to 0.0604 cm.

The heat exchange rate between blood and the surroundings can be calculated from

(5.3) $WC_P(T_{out} - T_{in}) = UA\left[\dfrac{(T_s - T_{out}) - (T_s - T_{in})}{2.3 \log (T_s - T_{out})/(T_s - T_{in})}\right]$

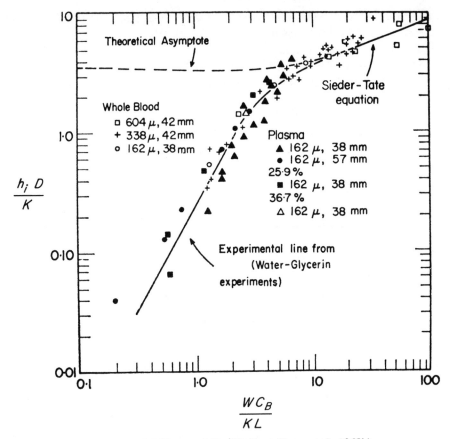

Fig. 5.3   Plot of h_iD/K versus WC_B/KL (from Charm et al., 1968b).

where $1/UA$ = overall resistance between surroundings and bulk of blood
U = overall heat transfer coefficient based on surface area A
A = surface area
T_s = surroundings temperature
T_{in} = inlet temperature of blood or suspension
T_{out} = outlet temperature of blood or suspension

The total or overall resistance is related to the resistance of the blood by

$$(5.4) \quad R_{total} = R_{(surroundings)} + R_{(vessel\ wall)} + R_{(blood)}$$

or

$$\frac{1}{UA} = \frac{1}{h_0 A_0} + \frac{X_w}{k_w A_m} + \frac{1}{h_i A_i}$$

where h_0 = heat transfer coefficient for surroundings (see Table 5.1 for some typical coefficients)

X_w = thickness of vessel wall

k_w = thermal conductivity of vessel wall

h_i = blood heat transfer coefficient

A_i = lateral surface area inside vessel

A_0 = surface area on outside of vessel wall

A_m = mean surface area of vessel (for thin walls this can be taken as equal to the inside or outside area)

Table 5.1   Estimates of Common "Surroundings" Heat Transfer Coefficients

Condition	h_0 (in units of) cal/[sec $(°C)(cm^2)$]
Still water	1.36×10^{-3}
Still air	1.36×10^{-4}
Rapidly moving air	5.45×10^{-4}
Rapidly flowing water	6.80×10^{-3}

When a thin-walled vessel or cylinder exists with $A_0 = A_i = A_m$, equation 5.4 becomes

$$(5.5) \quad \frac{1}{U} = \frac{1}{h_0} + \frac{X_w}{k_w} + \frac{1}{h_i}$$

Since temperature differences between surroundings and blood are usually small under physiological conditions when no marginal plasma layer exists, $\mu_w/K_B{}^2 = 1$, and the blood viscosity affects fluid heat transfer resistance only through its effect on flow rate W.

When still air is the surrounding medium, the effect of blood resistance is small compared with still air resistance. If water were the surrounding medium, however, blood resistance would be in the same order as water resistance (see Example 5.1).

Since heat transfers in the direction of a temperature gradient, heat cannot be removed from organs and tissue unless both are at a higher temperature than the blood, as indicated in equation 5.3.

5.2   EFFECT OF VISCOSITY ON MASS TRANSFER

Transfer resistance of a solute to and from fluids is influenced by the fluid viscosity and sometimes by fluid velocity. Since mass transfer occurs primarily in capillaries, plasma viscosity rather than blood viscosity is of main importance.

There is some evidence that capillaries are not the sole site of exchange (Majno et al., 1967). Using a miniaturized oxygen electrode having a tip diameter of 1μ (Whalen et al., 1967), it has been shown that tissue oxygen in the vicinity of arterioles is very nearly identical to the intraarteriolar pO_2 and that significant amounts of oxygen may leave the blood before it reaches the capillary bed (Duling and Berne, 1970).

Applying the classical "two-film model" (Lewis and Whitman, 1924) for mass transfer, the transfer of solute from a cell phase to a plasma phase entails passage through resistances associated with the cell phase and with the plasma phase (see Fig. 5.4). Concentration gradients, which exist across resistances to mass transfer, are analogous to the temperature gradients across resistances to heat transfer.

The rate of transfer of a solute from the bulk cell phase to the interface between the two phases is

$$(5.6) \quad \frac{dX}{dt} = K_x A(X - X_i)$$

where dX/dt = transfer rate through cell phase solute per unit of solute-free cell phase

X_i = (amount of solute at interface associated with cell phase)/(unit amount of solute free cell phase)

$1/K_x A$ = resistance associated with cell phase

A = exchange surface area

X = (amount of solute in bulk cell phase)/(unit amount of solute free cell phase)

K_x = mass transfer coefficient associated with cell phase

When the solute next passes from the interface through the resistance associated with the plasma phase, the rate of transfer is

$$(5.7) \quad \frac{dY}{dt} = K_y A(Y_i - Y)$$

where K_y = mass transfer coefficient associated with plasma phase

$1/K_y A$ = resistance associated with plasma phase

Y = (amount of solute in bulk plasma phase)/(unit amount of solute-free cell phase)

Y_i = (concentration of solute at interface associated with plasma phase)/(unit amount of solute-free plasma phase)

dY/dt = rate of solute transfer through plasma phase

At the interface, the solute in the plasma phase is in equilibrium with the solute in the cell phase, and we have

$$(5.8) \quad X_i = f(Y_i)$$

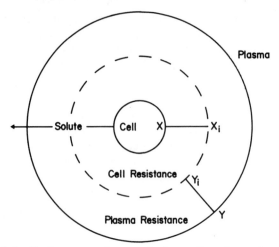

Fig. 5.4   Resistance to solute transfer from cell to plasma phase.

(This relationship can be determined experimentally by observing the relative amounts of solute in the plasma and cell phases after they have come to equilibrium.)

Since there is no accumulation of solute at the interface, we can write

$$(5.9) \quad \frac{dY}{dt} = \frac{dX}{dt}$$

Not infrequently one of the two resistances is controlling with respect to solute transfer. If the plasma phase is controlling, the viscosity of plasma affects the value of K_y.

In general, in a capillary, it is expected that

$$K_y = f(V, D_i, \mu_p, \rho, L, D, D_c, \phi)$$

where V = cell velocity relative to plasma velocity
        D_i = diffusion coefficient for solute
        μ_p = viscosity of plasma
        ρ = density of plasma
        L = length of capillary
        D = diameter of capillary
        D_c = cell diameter
        ϕ = cell volume fraction in capillary

The diffusion constant is related to viscosity (see, e.g., Glasstone, 1946) by

$$D_i = \frac{RT}{6\pi\mu_p aN}$$

where R = gas constant

$\quad T$ = absolute temperature

$\quad a$ = solute radius

$\quad N$ = Avogadro's number

The diffusion constant for oxygen in blood at $\phi = 0.45$ and $37°C$ is 1.24×10^{-5} cm^2/sec; in plasma it is 1.8×10^{-5} cm^2/sec (Stein et al., 1971).

From oxygen transfer data in the lung, we can calculate the diffusion coefficient to be 1.16×10^{-7} cm^2/sec (see Example 5.2). The discrepancy between this value and that obtained by Stein suggests that oxygen transfer in the lung is not a true diffusion process. The relative role of intracellular diffusive and convective oxygen transport in red cell suspension has been studied by subjecting the suspension to viscometric flow in a cone and plate viscometer and measuring the initial release of oxygen with a mass spectrophotometer. The results showed that in flowing red cells, the convection of oxygen and oxyhemoglobin is of greater significance than diffusion (Zander and Schmid-Schönbein, 1972).

Through dimensional analysis it would be possible to reduce these variables to dimensionless groups that could be correlated experimentally. If there are nine variables capable of being expressed in three fundamental dimensions (mass, length, and time), there will be six dimensionless groups (e.g., Brown, 1960). In this case, suitable dimensionless groups are

$$\underset{\text{I}}{\frac{K_y}{(D_i)D}} = f \underset{\text{II}}{\frac{(D_i)D}{V}}, \quad \underset{\text{II}}{\frac{\mu_p}{(D_i)}}, \quad \underset{\text{III}}{\frac{L}{D}}, \quad \underset{\text{IV}}{\frac{Dc}{D}}, \quad \underset{\text{V}}{\phi}$$

By varying each group separately and holding others constant, $K_y/(D_i)D$ can be related to the dimensionless groups experimentally. By varying V and evaluating $K_y/(D_i)D$, it would be possible to design experiments holding groups II, III, IV, V constant while group I is varied.

Roughton (1963) has considered the transfer of carbon dioxide and carbon monoxide in red cell suspensions. He notes that the uptake rate of oxygen by hemoglobin is decreased as the viscosity of the suspending medium increases. There have been no experiments yet in which the mass transfer coefficients are evaluated as a function of plasma viscosity.

Either the cell phase or the plasma phase may control the rate of transfer of a solute from a red cell to plasma, owing to the relatively high resistance of each phase to the solute transfer. If the plasma phase controls, the whole concentration gradient occurs across the resistance associated with the plasma phase – that is, from the interface to the bulk plasma phase (see Fig. 5.4). There is no concentration gradient between the cell phase and the interface.

When solute is transferred in a steady state from one phase to another in a

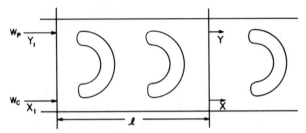

Fig. 5.5   Solute transfer along length of capillary.

given length of capillary, it is possible to relate concentrations along the length by a solute material balance, as in Fig. 5.5. The material balance results in

$$(5.10) \quad W_P(Y_1 - Y) = W_c(X_1 - X) = \frac{dY}{dt} = \frac{dX}{dt} = W_p \, dY = W_c \, dX$$

where W_p = mass flow rate of solute-free plasma
    W_c = mass flow rate of solute-free cell
    X_1 = (solute in cell phase)/(cell phase less solute) at entrance to capillary
    Y_1 = (solute in plasma phase)/(cell phase less solute) at entrance to capillary
    X = (solute of cell phase)/(cell phase less solute) at capillary cross section a distance from entrance
    Y = (solute in plasma phase)/(cell phase less solute) at capillary cross section a distance from entrance

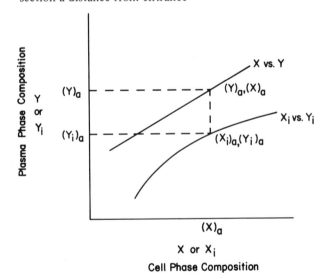

Fig. 5.6   Mass balance relationship between Y and X and equilibrium relationships between X_i and Y_i.

As Fig. 5.6 indicates, equation 5.10 can be plotted; that is, if W_p, W_c, X_1, and Y_1 are known, Y can be treated as a function of X. Equation 5.8 can be plotted similarly [i.e., $X_i = f(Y_i)$ – see Fig. 5.6].

The exchange surface area A can be expressed by

(5.11) $A = as\,dl$

where s = cross-sectional area

a = transfer area per unit volume in capillary

dl = differential length

Rearranging equation 5.7 and substituting equation 5.11 for A, we obtain

(5.12) $$\int_{Y_i}^{Y} \frac{dY}{Y_i - Y} = \frac{K_y as}{W_p} \int_{l_1}^{l} dl = \frac{K_y as(l - l_1)}{W_p}$$

If the plasma phase transfer is controlling and K_y is the controlling mass transfer coefficient, equation 5.12 expresses the solute concentration in the plasma phase in a capillary cross section as a function of distance l along the length of the capillary.

Equation 5.12 is solved graphically using Fig. 5.6. This is done by plotting $1/(Y_i - Y)$ versus Y (see Fig. 5.7). To find Y_i for any $Y = (Y)_a$, select a corresponding value of $X = (X)_a$ from the Y versus X curve. Since the plasma phase or K_y is controlling, there is no concentration gradient across the X or cell phase resistance, and the bulk concentration of the X phase $(X)_a$ is equal to the interface concentration associated with the X phase; that is $(X_i)_a$. Since $(X)_a = (X_i)_a$, $(X_i)_a$ is known from the X_i versus Y_i curve in Fig. 5.6; thus $(Y_i)_a$ is found from the same plot. Consequently $1/[(Y_i)_a - Y_a]$ can be evaluated for $Y = Y_a$.

The plot of $1/(Y_i - Y)$ versus Y is determined in the following manner (see Fig. 5.7). As equation 5.12 indicates, the area under the curve is K_y as $(l_2 - l_1)$. Knowing K_y as, it is possible to find l as a function of Y by taking various areas under the curve and solving for l. If concentrations of solute are known along the length of a capillary, K_y can be evaluated by reversing the procedure.

In the case of oxygen transfer from lung alveoli to hemoglobin in blood, the blood phase is the phase-controlling gas exchange as compared with the alveolar phase (e.g., Riley, 1965). Krogh (1919) proposed a simple model in which the diffusion of oxygen in tissue controlled oxygenation. However, work of Roughton and Forster (1957) indicates that intracapillary oxygen transfer may dictate the limiting rate at which oxygen can be supplied to the adjoining tissues.

A plot of the equilibrium relationship between partial pressure of oxygen and (moles of O_2)/moles of O_2-free hemoglobin) appears in Fig. 5.8. Using this information, the mass transfer coefficient is calculated to be $K_y = 2.59 \times 10^{-9}$ moles HHb/(sec) (cm^2), (see Example 5.2). With this value and assuming a

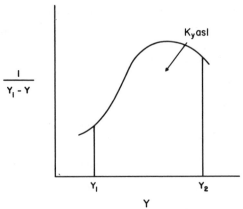

Fig. 5.7   Graphical solution for $dR/Y = Kasl.$

capillary diameter of 1.0×10^{-3} cm, we determine that the time for blood in the lung to reach 98% of its equilibrium value with respect to oxygen is about 0.25 sec.

It has been mathematically demonstrated that convection due to plasma bolus eddies does not contribute significantly to the transfer of oxygen and other dissolved gases in the circulation, (Aroesty and Gross, 1969).

Convection due to eddies plays a significant role in overall species transport only if the Peclet number v_c/D_iX is greater than 10 (v_c is cell velocity, X is distance between cells, and D_i is the diffusion coefficient for species in the space between erythrocytes).

However, the transport of slowly diffusing, high molecular weight materials (e.g., proteins) may be influenced by plasma bolus eddies even if they have Peclet numbers greater than 10 (Aroesty and Gross).

Example 5.1

A man walking at 3.0 mph has a metabolic rate of 130 kcal/(hr)(m²) (Adams and Iampietro, 1968). How much of this heat is removed by convection and radiation to surroundings at 25°C?

Given

thermal conductivity of blood $k_B = 1.24 \times 10^{-3}$ cal-cm/(sec)(°C)(cm²)

specific heat of blood $C_P = 0.98$ cal/(g)(°C)

skin thickness $X_w = 0.2$ cm

heat transfer coefficient for still air $h_0 = 1.36 \times 10^{-4}$ cal/(sec)(cm²)(°C)

skin thermal conductivity $= 1.23 \times 10^{-3}$ cal-cm/(sec)(°C)(cm²)

heat transfer coefficient for radiant heat transfer

(Ruch and Patton, 1965) $= 1.95 \times 10^{-4}$ cal/(sec)(cm²)(sec)

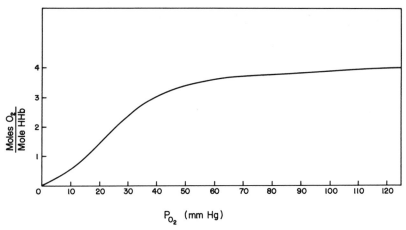

Fig. 5.8   Equilibrium relationship for partial pressure of oxygen and hemoglobin in blood.

$$\text{skin emissivity (average black and white)} = 0.75$$
$$\text{capillary length} = 0.1 \text{ cm}$$
$$\text{capillary diameter} = 10^{-3} \text{ cm}$$
$$\text{volume flow rate in capillary} = 5 \times 10^{-7} \text{ cm}^3/\text{sec}$$

Solution

The blood heat transfer coefficient inside a capillary is

$$\frac{h_i(10^{-3})}{1.24 \times 10^{-3}} = f \; \frac{5 \times 10^{-7} \times 0.98}{1.24 \times 10^{-3} \times 10^{-1}} \; f(4 \times 10^{-3})$$

Extrapolating in Fig. 5.3 gives $hD/K = 1.65 \times 10^{-3}$ and $h_i = 2.04 \times 10^{-3}$ cal/(sec)(cm^2)($^\circ$C).

The overall heat transfer coefficient U is found from equation 5.5:

$$\frac{1}{U} = \frac{1}{2.04 \times 10^{-3}} + \frac{0.2}{1.23 \times 10^{-3}} + \frac{1}{1.36 \times 10^{-4} + 0.75 \times 1.94 \times 10^{-4}}$$

$$U = 2.42 \times 10^{-4} \text{ cal/(sec)(cm}^2)(^\circ\text{C})$$

The rate of heat transfer per unit area is

$$Q = 2.42 \times 10^{-4}(37 - 25) = 29 \times 10^{-4} \text{ cal/(sec)(cm}^2)$$

or

$$106 \text{ kcal/(hr)(m}^2)$$

The fraction of metabolic heat removed by convection and radiation is

$$\frac{106}{130} = 0.82 \quad \text{or} \quad 82\%$$

The remaining heat is removed by evaporative cooling from skin and lungs.

The conclusion from this analysis is that the resistance to heat transfer by blood in capillaries is minor (10%) compared with the resistance offered by still air, which limits the rate of heat transfer in this case. If water were the surrounding medium, h_0 would be greater and the blood resistance would be of the same order as the surrounding resistance.

Winslow and Herrington (1949) suggest that 79% of metabolic heat is removed by radiation and convection and 21% by evaporative cooling. This is in good agreement with the results calculated here.

Example 5.2a

Determine the mass transfer coefficient for oxygen passing from alveoli in the lung to hemoglobin in blood. There is essentially no resistance to oxygen transfer from alveoli through the capillary wall. Blood phase resistance controls transfer of oxygen to hemoglobin.

Given

mole % O_2 in inspired air   = 21
mole % O_2 in expired air   = 16.5
surface area for transfer in lung   = 2×10^5 cm^2
    (assuming half capillaries are closed at any time)
blood flow rate   = 100 ml/sec
hemoglobin (HHb)   = 15 g/100 ml of blood
molecular weight of hemoglobin   = 66,800
flow rate of hemoglobin   = 2.25×10^{-4} moles/sec
pO_2 entering blood   = 40 mm Hg

Solution

pO_2 *in alveoli.* Inspired air is assumed to have 47 mm Hg water vapor partial pressure or a dry gas partial pressure of $760 - 47 = 713$ mm Hg. The partial pressure of oxygen in $0.21(713) = 150$ mm Hg (neglecting pressure loss due to lung air passage friction). Expired air is at atmospheric pressure, and the partial pressure of oxygen in $0.165(713) = 117$ mm Hg.

The average alveoli pO_2 between inspiration and expiration is 134 mm Hg. The equilibrium relationship between pO_2 in alveoli and oxygen in blood is given by Fig. 5.8.

The oxygen in blood is essentially all bound with hemoglobin (except for that dissolved in plasma). Therefore, Fig. 5.8 is the equilibrium relationship between oxygen in blood hemoglobin and oxygen in alveoli for various partial pressures. Let

$$Y = \frac{\text{moles of } O_2}{\text{mole of } O_2\text{-free HHb}} \qquad \text{in blood phase}$$

$$Y_i = \frac{\text{moles of } O_2}{\text{mole of } O_2\text{-free HHb}} \qquad \text{at blood-phase–alveoli-phase interface}$$

Equilibrium at pO_2 = 134 mm Hg gives the interface concentration of moles O_2/mole HHb or Y_i = 4.0 (see Fig. 5.8). At the capillary entrance with a blood pO_2 of 40 mm Hg, Y_1 = 3.0. At capillary exit, blood pO_2 = 100 mm Hg and Y_2 = 3.9.

The mass transfer coefficient is related to oxygen concentration by equation 5.12:

$$G \, dY = K \, dA \, (Y_i - Y) \qquad \text{or} \qquad \int_{Y_1}^{Y_2} \frac{dY}{Y_i - Y} = \frac{KA}{G}$$

where G = (oxygen-free hemoglobin) flow rate (moles/sec)

A = transfer surface area

Since Y_i is constant throughout area A, we have

$$(5.13) \quad \ln \frac{Y_i - Y_1}{Y_i - Y_2} = \frac{KA}{G}$$

Hence

$$\ln \frac{4.0 - 3.0}{4.0 - 3.9} = \frac{K(2.0 \times 10^5)}{2.25 \times 10^{-4}}$$

$$K = 2.59 \times 10^{-9} \text{ moles HHb/(sec)(cm}^2\text{)}$$

The mass transfer coefficient K, although determined from consideration of the total exchange area of the lung, also applies to transfer in individual capillaries. This coefficient may be a function of velocity. Over the relatively narrow range of flow associated with the lung, however, it is not expected that K will vary greatly (e.g., Middleman, 1972). In addition, the transfer coefficient is affected by the viscosity of both the plasma and the cell contents in a manner that has not yet been quantitated.

Example 5.2b

Using the mass transfer coefficient calculated in Example 5.2a, calculate how oxygen concentration varies along the length of a capillary and determine how long is required for hemoglobin to come to 98% equilibrium with the oxygen in the alveoli.

Solution

The available surface area for oxygen transfer is 2×10^5 cm^2. With $D = 1 \times 10^{-3}$ cm and $L = 0.1$ cm, the number of capillaries with cells flowing is

$$N(\pi DL) = 2 \times 10^5 \qquad \text{or} \qquad N = 0.64 \times 10^9 \text{ capillaries}$$

The hemoglobin flow rate per capillary is

$$\frac{2.25 \times 10^{-4}}{0.64 \times 10^9} = 3.50 \times 10^{-13} \text{ moles/sec}$$

The exchange surface area for a capillary is also πDl, where l is the distance along the capillary measured from the entrance. Thus from Example 5.2a we have

$$\frac{Y_i - Y_1}{Y_i - Y} = e^{KA/G}$$

where $Y_i = 4.0$
$\quad Y_1 = 3.0$
$\quad K = 2.59 \times 10^{-9}$ moles HHb/(sec)(cm^2)
$\quad G = 3.5 \times 10^{-13}$ moles HHb/sec (for a capillary)
$\quad D = 1 \times 10^{-3}$ cm

The oxygen concentration as a function of distance along the capillary is $Y = 4.0 \, l^{-23.3l}$.

When $l = 0.1$ cm, which is the end of the capillary, $Y = 4 - 0.097 = 3.903$. Thus oxygen concentration is 97.5%.

Time to Reach 97.5% of Equilibrium Concentration

There are 0.64×10^9 open capillaries in the lung, their average diameter being 1×10^{-3} cm, and since the flow rate through the lung is 100 ml/sec, the flow rate through a capillary is $100/(0.64 \times 10^9) = 3.1 \times 10^{-7}$ cm^3/sec. Thus the velocity must be

$$\frac{3.1 \times 10^{-7}}{\pi/4(1 \times 10^{-3})} = 0.4 \text{ cm/sec}$$

The time to travel 0.1 cm, therefore, is 0.25 sec. This is the time required to reach 97.5% of equilibrium concentration.

A model describing oxygen transfer across the placenta between parallel capillaries, in which the resistance offered by the intracellular hemoglobin reaction is considered, predicts that pO_2 reaches 99.4% equilibration by the end of a 1.7-sec capillary transit (Hill et al., 1972).

5.3 DIFFUSION COEFFICIENT FOR OXYGEN TRANSFER IN THE LUNGS IF TRANSFER OCCURS THROUGH A DIFFUSION PROCESS

The mass transfer equation often appears with concentration expressed in terms of volume (e.g., moles O_2/cm^3) rather than in moles of inert material (e.g., moles O_2/moles O_2-free hemoglobin), as it has been employed in the previous section.

The units of the mass transfer coefficient depend on the way concentration is expressed. In equation 5.12, for example, the units of the mass transfer coefficient are determined by substituting the units for the various symbols; that is,

$$W_p \, dY = K_y A \, dl$$

$$\frac{\text{moles inert}}{\text{sec}} \cdot \frac{\text{moles solute}}{\text{moles inert}} = K_y \cdot \text{cm}^2 \cdot \frac{\text{moles solute}}{\text{moles inert}}$$

$$\frac{1}{\text{sec/cm}^2} = K_y$$

Concentration can be converted from moles/mole inert to moles/cm³ by multiplying moles/mole inert by moles inert/cm³.

Thus, substituting again in equation 5.12, we obtain

$$\frac{\text{moles inert}}{\text{cm}^3} \cdot \frac{\text{moles inert}}{\text{sec}} \cdot \frac{\text{moles solute}}{\text{moles inert}} = K_y{}^1 \cdot \text{cm}^2 \cdot \frac{\text{moles inert}}{\text{cm}^3} \cdot \frac{\text{moles solute}}{\text{moles inert}}$$

and

$$\frac{\text{cm}}{\text{sec}} = K_y{}^1 \qquad \text{or} \qquad K_y \frac{\text{moles inert}}{\text{cm}^3} = K_y{}^1$$

It is sometimes necessary to convert mass transfer coefficient units in order to make a comparison, as shown in the following computations. In blood, there are 2.24×10^{-6} moles HHb/cm³.

$$K^1 = \frac{2.59 \times 10^{-9}}{2.24 \times 10^{-6}} = 1.16 \times 10^{-3} \text{ cm}^3/(\text{sec})(\text{cm}^2)$$

$$D_i \cong 1.16 \times 10^{-7} \text{ cm}^2/\text{sec}$$

Assume that mass transfer in the lung occurs as a pure diffusion process such that $D_i \Delta c/\Delta T = K^1 \Delta c$ or $D_i/\Delta T = K^1$, where D_i is the diffusion constant and ΔT

the layer thickness over which the oxygen driving force acts (i.e., the average difference in oxygen concentration between alveoli and blood Δc). It is then possible to estimate a value for the diffusion constant for oxygen in blood.

Thus $D_i/\Delta T = 1.16 \times 10^{-3}$, and assuming that ΔT is in the order of 10^{-4} cm (i.e., capillary wall thickness), we have

$$D_i \cong 1.16 \times 10^{-7} \text{ cm}^2/\text{sec}$$

However, it was previously noted that the diffusion coefficient for oxygen in blood is 1.24×10^{-5} cm^2/sec (Stein et al., 1971). The discrepancy occurs because oxygen transfer in the lung is not a simple diffusion process, and the estimated transfer thickness is of the order of 10^{-2} cm rather than 10^{-4} cm. It is unlikely that the transfer distance could be 10 times the diameter of the capillary.

5.4   TRANSFER TO TISSUE

The model considered for calculating the rate of oxygen transfer from alveolar space to blood assumed that the rate of reaction complexing oxygen with hemoglobin is very rapid as compared with the mass transfer rate to the hemoglobin.

The transfer of oxygen and other solutes from capillaries to tissue in the presence of a metabolic reaction rate in the tissue has been reviewed and analyzed by Middleman (1972). The models employ the Krogh cylinder concept of arranging tissue with capillary; that is, a cylinder of tissue surrounding a capillary is the volume to which material is transferred from the capillary.

Blum (1960) considered transfer of a solute to tissue in the presence of a first-order chemical reaction. It is observed that the average capillary velocity plays a dominant role among the physiological variables appearing in the equation (Middleman, 1972).

An analytical solution is presented for the case of a steady-state metabolic rate for radial diffusion through tissue by Blum:

$$(5.14) \quad c = c_a + \frac{g_o}{D_r} \left[\frac{R^2 - R_a^2}{4} - \frac{R_t}{2} \ln \frac{R}{R_a} - \frac{g_o}{\bar{v}} \left(\frac{R_t^2}{R_a^2} - 1 \right) l \right]$$

where C_a = inlet oxygen concentration

R_a = radius of capillary

R_t = radius of tissue cylinder (i.e., measured from axis of capillary to point at which no oxygen flux exists in tissue)

R = distance from capillary axis

g_o = metabolic rate for tissue consumption of oxygen

$\bar{v}$ = average capillary velocity

D_r = diffusion constant for oxygen in tissue (assumed to be the same for blood)

Within the capillary, average oxygen concentration falls linearly with distance from the entrance, as shown by

$$(5.15) \quad c = c_a - \frac{g_o}{\bar{v}} \left(\frac{R_t^2}{R_c^2} - 1 \right) l$$

The dependence on velocity is much weaker in the case of constant metabolic rate than for a first-order metabolic rate. It is concluded that equations 5.14 and 5.15 give good approximations to oxygen profiles in the Krogh cylinder as long as oxygen consumption is constant throughout the tissue, that is, zero-order reaction or independent of concentration (Middleman, 1972). It is also indicated that neglect of axial diffusion in the capillary leads to significant errors unless the Peclet number $R_a \bar{v}/Dr$ is much greater than 1. For typical capillary conditions, Middleman points out that the Peclet number is 2.5, which indicates that neglect of axial diffusion introduces some error; the ease of analysis often justifies the approximation, however.

Employing equation 5.15 with the following values, Middleman calculated the oxygen concentration within a capillary as a function of distance along the length: $R_a = 3 \mu$, $R_t = 30 \mu$, $L = 180 \mu$, $P_A = 28.5$ mm Hg, $v = 400 \mu$/sec, $g_o = 0.85 \times 10^{-3}$ ml of oxygen/(ml)(sec), and $D_r = 1700 \mu^2$/sec. At the capillary entrance P_A is 28.5 mm Hg.

Figure 5.8 shows that blood is 55% saturated and with $0.2(0.55) = 0.11$ ml of oxygen/ml of blood. At a point midway along the capillary (i.e., $l = 90 \mu$), c is found from equation 5.15 as follows:

$$\dot{c} = 0.11 - 0.85 \times 10^{-3} \; [10^2 - 1] \; 90 = 0.091 \text{ ml O}_2/\text{ml blood}$$

Thus the percentage of saturation $0.091/0.2 = 0.455$, and employing Fig. 5.8 it is determined that this corresponds to $pO_2 = 24$ mm Hg. Similarly, at $l = 180 \mu$, there is 36% saturation and the pO_2 is 20 mm Hg.

Oxygen tension in the tissue was calculated taking $r = 16.5 \mu$ and using equation 5.14 at $l = 0$, $P_{tissue} = 17$ mm Hg; at $l = 180 \mu$, P_{tissue} was 8.5 mm Hg.

Viscosity in Clinical Medicine

Chapter 6

6.1 STATE OF THE ART

IN THE PREVIOUS CHAPTERS WE HAVE OUTLINED the factors controlling flow in the microcirculation. These included (1) the geometric and functional characteristics of the circulation — the length, diameter, and taper of the vessel; the nature of the vessel wall: its elasticity and endothelial lining, and the velocity of flow; and (2) the characteristics of the flowing suspension — the number of cells; their shape, size, and rigidity; and the nature of the suspending medium, including its protein and fat contents. In this chapter we consider some of the clinical implications of these phenomena.

Before turning to clinical states in which alteration of blood viscosity appears to play a role, it is well to recognize the limitations of our present knowledge. No suitable intravascular viscometer has yet been devised; despite efforts to attack the problem (Frasher et al., 1969) we remain ignorant of the rheology of blood in its native environment. Determinations in our best viscometers may be subject to artifact, moreover, and the errors in our present simplifying assumptions may be of an order of magnitude that limits conclusions.

A few examples serve to illustrate these problems. Viscometers that operate at high shear rates give information about asymptotic viscosity but tell little about properties at low shear rates, which may be more relevant in parts of the microcirculation. Blood in a low shear rate cone and plate viscometer (below $1 \sec^{-1}$) begins to separate as soon as it is added (Schmid-Schönbein et al., 1971b). Furthermore, in experiments in which flow in a living vessel has been compared to that anticipated on the basis of formulas devised for glass capillaries, the energy losses *in vivo* have been unexpectedly low (Djojosugito et al., 1970; Skovborg et al., 1968; Kurland et al., 1966; Whitaker and Winton, 1933; Levy and Share, 1953). No satisfactory explanation is yet available, but hypotheses implicate the elasticity of the wall, electrical charges across the wall, and the nature of the endothelial lining. For example, Copley (1960) has suggested that wall adherence of plasma serum is less in contact with a surface of fibrin than with glass. Djojosugito et al., felt that the discrepancies between blood viscosity *in vivo* and *in vitro* were related to vascular dimensions favoring bolus flow. On the other hand, Benis et al., (1970) studied pressure–flow relations in the hind paw of the dog and concluded that a flow curve corrected for inertial effects was indistinguishable from the viscometric one, (See Section 3.3).

Further difficulty arises from lack of knowledge of the functional geometry of the microvasculature in man (Burton, 1966; Sobin and Tremer, 1966) and from its heterogeneity. Data on flowing blood are available only in limited circulations in animals based on the ability to transilluminate the structure — for example, the hamster's cheek pouch (Fulton et al., 1946; Greenblatt et al., 1969), the bat's wing (Wiedeman, 1963), the mesentery of rats (Zweifach, 1961) and frogs (Bloch, 1962), and the atria of cats (Tillich et al., 1971; Hellberg et al.,

1972). Only the surface of solid organs such as lung or liver has been readily available. Studies deeper in solid organs produce trauma in the subject. The relevance of studies in thin tissue to blocks has been questioned (Lamport, 1964). The data in man, which are even more fragmentary, consist largely of visualization of the nail beds and the bulbar conjunctivae under strong light (Bloch, 1959; Wells, 1966) and the vessels of the mesentery at the time of abdominal surgery (Guest, 1971). A titanium chamber has been implanted in a twin-pedicled skin tube in man to extend the scope of investigation (Branemark, 1963). The use of chamber techniques to study the microvasculature has been reviewed by Nims and Irwin (1973).

The geometry of the circulation has been established in animals by quick freezing (Phibbs, 1966, 1967), radioopaque injection, and microvascular casting techniques; but again, data in man are limited (Lundskog et al., 1968). Moreover, inadequate attention has been paid to the heterogeneity of the circulation in different organs. Note the special circulations in the kidney and lung, as well as differences in the tapering of small arteries and the angle of branching. For example, medullary flow in the dog's kidney is viscosity dependent but cortical flow is independent (Nashat et al., 1964). Of great importance, finally, is our limited knowledge of shear rates in the circulations of human organs. For example, Whitmore (1968) estimates mean shear rates at $40 \sec^{-1}$ in the venae cavae and higher in other organs, whereas others speculate on values as low as 0 to $20 \sec^{-1}$ (Wells, 1962; Merrill et al., 1963). These differences may be critical, since the rate of shear in the microcirculation is the disruptive force that tends to disperse aggregates (Schmid-Schönbein, 1968).

Despite these limitations in our knowledge, considerable insight into the function of the microcirculation has been attained (Johnson, 1972). The quantitative methods outlined in previous chapters provide a framework to which new data can be applied as they become available.

As we see below, the tendency to form aggregates is enhanced in a variety of conditions, some characterized by rises in plasma fibrinogen or other macromolecules, others by presumed changes in the red cell membrane (Thorsen and Hint, 1950); in still others, the phenomenon is the result of mechanisms not yet elucidated. The response of the body to cellular aggregation is only poorly understood. An extensive review of "sludging," the intravascular aggregation of erythrocytes into wads and masses, has been provided by Knisely (1965), who believes that aggregation is not seen in normal man and animal. Others have suggested that aggregates form normally (Ditzel, 1959; Robertson et al., 1950) but are easily reversed as shear increases. In contrast, aggregates in sick patients appear to be more firmly bound (Schmid-Schönbein, 1971b; Goldstone et al., 1970). The response of the body to the formation of large numbers of aggregates depends on their number and size and on the balance between the forces binding and fragmenting them. Aggregates may obstruct flow at the capillary entrance, or they may disperse, only to reform on the venous side (Berman, 1962). In the event of obstruction of capillaries, tissue flow may be maintained by the opening of other capillary pathways or arteriovenous shunts. The response of the microcirculation to aggregate formation is further complicated by the vasomotor response, which sometimes includes prolonged vasoconstriction (Rosenblum, 1969).

When extensive aggregation has been produced experimentally, as by high molecular weight dextran or antisera, a variety of hemodynamic phenomena have been described: increased vascular resistance and a rise in the critical closing pressure (Hint, 1964), decreased cardiac output (Gelin et al., 1968), as well as interference in flow and resultant hypoxic damage (Stalker, 1964). With intermittent plugging, flow stops but pressure remains high and aggregates increase in size (Bloch et al., 1961, 1965). The extent to which any of these phenomena occur in man can be visualized only to a limited extent in the bulbar circulation, where altered morphology, increased aggregation, and reduced velocity of flow can be observed in some states (Madow and Bloch, 1956; Wells, 1967).

On the other hand, in contrast to Knisely and Bloch, Pories et al., (1962) and Heimbecker and Bigelow (1950) have presented evidence suggesting that the bulbar conjunctivae are not valid samples of all arterial blood. Clinical knowledge of aggregate formation is vital to the application of the model of the microcirculation now widely accepted, which postulates that red cells exist in clumps or aggregates at very low or zero shear rates and that such clump formations are increasingly fractured until, at shear rates above a 100 sec^{-1}, blood has almost Newtonian properties. Efforts to estimate the extent of intravascular aggregation by simple *in vitro* tests have included use of the sedimentation rate and the screen filtration test (Swank et al., 1965). The use of the former method for this purpose has been criticized by Knisely (1965), and Davis and Woodliff (1966) found only a good general relationship between viscosity and sedimentation rate, with many individual differences. Dhall et al. (1969) have show that screen filtration pressure does not measure red cell aggregation.

Our discussion of viscosity in clinical states deals first with the concentration of red blood cells, then with the elasticity and other properties of the cells, and finally with the influence of plasma protein and fat.

6.2   EFFECT OF VOLUME FRACTION OF RED BLOOD CELLS AND VASCULAR DISEASE

Both the red-cell—red-cell attraction and the protein—red-cell interaction are a function of the red cell concentration, and both viscosity and yield stress increase as hematocrit increases. In fact, the volume fraction of red cells is the major determinant of viscosity. A mathematical expression for this relation has been described earlier (Chapter 2). However, as indicated, viscosity also varies inversely as the velocity or shear rate. Thus the classical picture of viscosity increasing moderately with hematocrit at low levels and rising sharply above 58% (Pirofsky, 1953; Mendlowitz, 1948) should be amended as illustrated by Wells (1961) to include a family of curves, each showing the inverse relation of viscosity to shear rate but rising most steeply at high hematocrits and low shear rates. As we have pointed out, the rate of shear at the wall of the vessels in the human circulation can only be estimated. Estimates vary from 100 to 200 sec^{-1} for the aorta to approximately 10 sec^{-1} or less for the venules. Clearly, however, in parts of the venous system and in small vessels, flow may be phasic and even occasionally reversed, and viscosity must reach very high levels with sharp increases in hematocrit. Consideration should also be given to the influence of hematocrit on the relatively cell-free area at the vessel wall in arterioles. Whatever the origin of this zone, which we have discussed earlier, its width is a function of the volume fraction of red blood cells and may be another means by which hematocrit influences flow in small vessels. The consequences of increased red cell volume fraction are also influenced by cell deformation (Chien et al., 1970; Schmid-Schönbein; et al., 1969; Weed, 1970). The shear thinning behavior of blood is especially marked at high hematocrits when cell collisions are increased. Here deformation of cells is a major factor in reducing viscosity and facilitating flow in minute vessels.

Significant elevation of blood hematocrit is found in polycythemia vera, secondary polycythemia, and erythremia. The incidence of thromboses in polycythemia vera, which is as high as 33% (Wasserman and Gilbert, 1966; Burris and Arrowsmith, 1953; Calabressi and Meyer, 1959), occurs in the coronary, cerebral (Millikan, 1960), pulmonary, and other vascular beds. The mechanisms of vascular occlusion in polycythemia include (a) the high viscosity and high yield stress caused by the high hematocrit, (b) a reduction in the velocity of blood flow (hence decrease in shear rate), and (c) local vascular disease. Moreover, flow is not retarded equally in all systems. In the areas of slowest flow and highest hematocrit, greatly increased relative viscosity must occur. In polycythemia, it has been postulated, occlusion in the coronary circulation is less frequent than elsewhere because of the absence of stagnation in the vessels of an actively contracting organ (Videbaek, 1950). Thromboses of large-calibre vessels are rare. The combination of uncontrolled erythremia and surgery is particularly hazardous and results in a high incidence of thrombosis or hemorrhage. Reduction of viscosity by reduction of hematocrit reduces the morbidity in surgery by a factor of 3 and the deaths by a factor of 7 (Wasserman and Gilbert, 1966). Hemodilution with hypertonic sodium chloride is accompanied by an increase in cardiac output and stroke volume without change in systemic blood pressure; there is also a decrease in peripheral and pulmonary vascular resistance (Rowe et al., 1972).

Secondary polycythemia is found in cyanotic heart disease, chronic lung disease, extreme obesity, metabolic diseases of the red blood cell, some forms of chronic renal disease, and a number of erythropoetin-producing tumors. The hemodynamic consequences of elevated hematocrit in these diseases, when not accompanied by a panmyelopathy, do not seem to be significantly different from those in polycythemia vera. Evidence of the clinical consequences derives from studies of persons living at high altitude (Balke, 1964). Indeed, the hematopoetic system is stimulated within hours of reaching high altitude. The hemoglobin content rises from 15.3 mg/100 ml at sea level to 24.8 g at 6500 m. Despite the great increase in viscosity, experience in mountaineering has shown that men with more than 8×10^6 red blood cells per milliliter of blood function well at altitudes of 7000 to 8000 m as long as weather is tolerable and dehydration is avoided. During severe cold and storms, when subjects experience inadequate fluid intake, however, rapid deterioration occurs; this has been ascribed to peripheral vasoconstriction and further increase of the already high viscosity due to dehydration. Moreover, excessive erythrocytosis occurs in some subjects, leading to an incapacitating illness (Monge's disease) with hematocrit readings at times in the 80% range. This abnormality is attributed to an inappropriately low response to a decrease of oxygen (Penaloza and Francesco, 1971; Hecht, 1971).

High viscosity has also been indicted as a cause of intestinal disturbances experienced at high altitude after normal meals. Such high viscosity might be expected to increase vascular resistance and produce elevation of blood pressure. However, studies among Andean miners revealed that the individuals with the highest hematocrit in fact had the lowest blood pressure (Talbott and Dill, 1936; Marticorena et al., 1969). It has been suggested that this phenomenon is due to an effective general vasodilation. Some confirmation of this hypothesis may be found in the increase vascularity of brain, heart, and muscle of polycythemic rats (Miller and Hale, 1970). The coagulability of blood at high altitude is not abnormal, nor is the incidence of coronary artery disease increased. In fact, fatal coronary occlusion is said to be less frequent in the Andes than at sea level (Hultgren and Grover, 1968).

Extensive experience has also been obtained from studies in neonates and in children with cyanotic congenital heart disease, two conditions in which extremely high whole blood viscosity is found. Spontaneous hematocrit determinations as high as 75% have been noted in the normal neonate, and these values have been associated with a relative viscosity of 24.4 cP at a shear rate of 11.5 sec^{-1} (Baum, 1966). However, extreme elevations of hematocrit have been found with surprising frequency in infants with neurological, cardiologic, or respiratory dysfunction. Cutaneous hematocrits between 77 and 95%, corresponding to venous hematocrit of 79%, have been recorded (Baum, 1967). Treatment by partial exchange transfusion with plasma (Baum, 1967; Replogle et al., 1967) and infusion of dextrose (Danks and Stevens, 1964) are measures that have decreased hematocrit and improved pH and pCO_2 factors which, if uncorrected, would further increase red cell rigidity and enhance viscosity (Giombi and Burnard, 1970).

In cyanotic congenital heart disease, increases in hematocrit above 75% are said to be associated with symptomatology (Rudolph et al., 1953). Since minor increases in hematocrit at these levels produce marked elevations in blood viscosity, venesection has been suggested to keep the hematocrit below 60% (Kontras, 1968). Acute reduction of viscosity and yield shear stress by removal of red cells and replacement with plasma results in improved blood flow and oxygen transport (Rosenthal et al., 1970). The combination of cyanotic heart disease, anoxia, and increased blood viscosity can produce ischemic brain lesions, providing favorable areas for anaerobic bacterial growth.

Increased viscosity of lesser degree is seen in the secondary polycythemia, which accompanies respiratory insufficiency and chronic cor pulmonale in the adult. In this circumstance, no clear guidelines have been formulated between the need to reduce viscosity (and thereby pulmonary vascular resistance) on the one hand and the need to maximize oxygen transport on the other (Mack and Snider, 1956). Evidence from populations living at high altitude suggests that if secondary polycythemia ceases to be advantageous as a result of increased viscosity, difficulty must occur at hematocrits above 60% (Hultgren and Grover, 1968). Repeated bleeding which prevented polycythemia in rats held at high altitude, permitted the same exercise performance as at sea level minimizing pathological changes (Aetland and Highman, 1971). Venesection in man returning hematocrit and viscosity to normal produces only a small average drop in pulmonary blood pressure at rest. Clinical improvement, however, is described as modest but appreciable (Segel and Bishop, 1966).

More recently, a third condition associated with an elevated hematocrit has attracted renewed attention. Gaisbock (1922) applied the term "polycythemia hypertonica" to a group of patients with elevated red blood cell counts and hypertension in whom he noted tendencies to arteriosclerosis, enlarged heart, "habitus apoplecticus," and sometimes strokes. Lawrence and Berlin (1952) found the red cell volume normal and the plasma volume reduced; they postulated an emotional origin, applying the term "stress polycythemia." Others have called the condition pseudopolycythemia or benign polycythemia (Hall, 1965; Russell and Conley, 1964). The hematocrit is between 55 and 60% and there are no abnormalities of platelets or white blood cells nor splenomegaly.

In a group of 20 such patients, 7 of them under 50 years of age, 10 demonstrated vascular disease in the heart or elsewhere (Hall, 1965). The data suggest that the incidence of vascular disease may be related to the height of the hematocrit and the state of the vessels rather than to the identity of the condition – primary polycythemia or pseudopolycythemia. On the other hand, a recent study of spurious (relative) polycythemia points out that several types of alteration in red cell and plasma volumes can account for the high hematocrit. The most common was a combination of high normal red cell mass with low normal plasma volume. Moreover, the subjects with high hematocrit value showed no increase in abnormal clinical features (Brown et al., 1971).

It is not clear whether the benign polycythemia syndrome can be clearly differentiated from the positive and significant correlation between hematocrit and diastolic blood pressure reported by McDonough et al. (1965). The tendency of hypertensive male subjects to have a higher hematocrit and whole blood viscosity than normal men has been confirmed by Tibblin et al. (1966). On exercise, a significant increase in hematocrit and whole blood viscosity has been found in both groups.

Burch and dePasquale (1961, 1962, 1963, 1965) coupled the observation of an increased incidence of coronary artery disease in this group with a reawakening interest in blood rheology. They noted that both male and female patients with myocardial infarction or angina pectoris had erythrocytosis and that their symptoms often improved after phlebotomy (1965). They cited also the decreased incidence of coronary thrombosis in patients with anemia, and the report from the Framingham study (Dawber, 1961) that high levels of hemoglobin are associated with an increase in the incidence of coronary artery disease. The mean hematocrit of 100 patients with acute myocardial infarction was found to be significantly higher than that of 100 control subjects.

Burch and dePasquale correlated the recorded increases of hematocrit with the well-known changes in coronary flow during the cardiac cycle and postulated marked increases in viscosity during the marked fall in flow in the coronary artery during systole, especially during isometric contraction (1965). They stressed, in addition, the decrease in linear flow rate proximal to an area of coronary arterial narrowing and the linear increase in yield stress with hematocrit. A decrease in the frequency of angina pectoris and an increase in the exercise tolerance followed phlebotomy in patients with ischemic heart disease and erythrocytosis. Their suggestion prompted an editorial on "phlebotomy, an ancient procedure turning modern" (*JAMA*, 1963).

However, Conley et al. (1964) compared the hematocrit values of three groups of normal men with those of 200 patients with myocardial infarction and found the mean hematocrit value of the patients to be slightly lower than that of each control group. Furthermore, the hematocrit values of a group of medical students showed no correlation with a history of coronary artery disease in the parents. The authors doubted the significance of hematocrit as a predisposing factor in acute myocardial infarction except at extremely high levels. Their doubts were shared by Vuopio and Eisalo (1964), Rosenblatt et al. (1965), and McDonough et al. (1965); yet Stables et al. (1967) found a hematocrit exceeding 48% in 51.5% of a group with myocardial infarction but in only 22.5% of control subjects, although the mean hematocrit of their control subjects was lower than that reported as normal for the altitude. The occurrence of elevated hematocrit during the first days of an acute myocardial infarction has been confirmed by Shillingford's group (Sedziwy, 1968), but its etiologic role is not clear. The subsequent fall in hematocrit may be due to fluid shifts (Sedziwy, 1968) but also to diagnostic venesection (Hershberg, 1972). Significantly, among the Bantu of Johannesburg, South Africa, vascular occlusion is extraordinarily rare despite the occurrence of high hematocrit, (Walker, 1963), and prognosis in patients with acute myocardial infarction is not related to hematocrit (Hershberg et al., 1972).

The difficulty in evaluating these conflicting views on the role of moderate hematocrit elevation in the etiology of vascular occlusion arises in part from the use of myocardial infarction as an end point. Myocardial infarction is only the most striking and visible complication of a largely subclinical disease of multifactorial origin — coronary atherosclerosis. A host of metabolic, genetic, and anatomic factors may far outweigh the importance of a change in viscosity arising from mild rises in hematocrit. Moreover, the changes in hematocrit may have considerable cardiovascular effects only partly related to the change in viscosity. Thus, for example, Zoll et al. (1961, 1952) demonstrated increased coronary collateral circulation in anemic pigs and humans, and their observations were confirmed by Eckstein (1955). Kattus (1959) suggested that the increased retrograde coronary flow in a case of reduced hematocrit was due to decreased viscosity. Very little information is available regarding coronary circulation in the presence of polycythemia vera. The expanded red cell mass has been associated with a considerable reduction in coronary blood flow (Gregg and Green, 1940) and increased oxygen extraction without change in oxygen usage. The relation of these changes to viscosity is not clear (Regan et al., 1960).

Striking physiologic changes in response to anemia have also been noted. In man and in the experimental animal, for example, there is an increase in venous return (Guyton and Richardson, 1961) and in cardiac output, which falls when hematocrit is restored (Richardson and Guyton, 1959). It has been demonstrated that the increase in cardiac output in acute experimental anemia occurs in response to a decrease in outflow impedance and an enhancement of myocardial contractility. The reduction in outflow impedance is determined by the decrease in whole blood viscosity (Murray et al., 1969). At the same time, as hematocrit falls there is a decrease in coronary artery resistance and an increase in coronary blood flow. In the normal animal, when the coronary vessels have been maximally dilated at a hematocrit of 24 to 31%, further anemia results in depression of left ventricular function. In the presence of coronary stenosis, dilatation cannot take place and depression of left ventricular function occurs with less anemia (Case et al., 1955). Despite the high myocardial flow in anemia, left ventricular oxygen uptake is decreased. A 50% increase in hematocrit in these cases markedly reduces coronary flow without change in oxygen consumption. Transfusion of normal dogs decreases myocardial flow and oxygen uptake with an increase of tension time index and contractility (Regan et al., 1963).

The findings just cited appear to be related to enhanced viscosity. The acute induction of polycythemia in normal dogs with resultant decrease in cardiac output seems to have metabolic significance leading to a rise in the lactate–pyruvate ratio; these changes are reversible with dilution (Replogle et al., 1967). In patients presenting chronic hypervolemia in polycythemia vera, the stroke volume and cardiac output are elevated with close correlation to the increased blood volume. Phlebotomy decreases stroke volume and cardiac output (Cobb et al., 1960). The effect of concentration on peripheral flow poses additional problems still only incompletely explored (Levy and Share, 1953; Benis et al., 1970; Rosenblum, 1970). Changes in vessel size, the non-Newtonian behavior of blood, inertial losses, changes in flow distribution, red cell deformation in small vessels, the Fahraeus-Lindquist effect, blood pressure changes, and changes in plasma viscosity all complicate an evaluation of flow changes due to hematocrit in experimental models.

A frequently posed clinical problem concerns the optimal hematocrit for a patient with coronary artery disease. It often presents itself in the following form: at what level should transfusion be performed in an anemic patient with angina or recent myocardial infarction? Where does the harm from loss of oxygen-carrying capacity exceed the benefit from improved flow resulting from decreased viscosity and impedance? Crowell et al. (1967) addressed the theory of this issue, and Example 2.2 sets forth some of the variables. Our own data suggest that the normal human hematocrit of 46% is optimal (see Example 2.2, page 56). Relevant also are the data of Case et al. (1955), suggesting that in the presence of coronary narrowing, deterioration of ventricular function occurs at a hematocrit well above the 24 to 31% level that is tolerable in normals. For this reason, we must view with caution the arguments demonstrating adequacy of oxygen transport, even with very low hemoglobin, in dogs with normal coronary vasculature (Replogle 1967). The precipitation of coronary insufficiency by severe anemia has been repeatedly observed in patients with atherosclerosis. Moreover, levels of anemia tolerated at rest may be poorly tolerated on effort. No rigid guidelines can yet be laid down, since the critical variable of the precise functional state of the coronary circulation cannot be clinically determined.

The presence of altered viscosity during an acute myocardial infarction has been studied by numerous investigators, yielding discordant results. Kellogg and Goodman (1960), Ditzel et al. (1968), and Karppinen (1970) noticed an increase in fibrinogen in patients with myocardial infarction and correlated this with an increase in plasma viscosity. An increase in whole blood viscosity was not noted initially but appeared in later determinations, especially in patients with moderate or severe infarctions. On the other hand, Langsjoen (1967) recorded increases with mild and moderate myocardial infarction but saw a progressive decrease in viscosity and hematocrit in severe cases, which he ascribed to aggregation and sequestration. Dintenfass (1963, 1964) studied the viscosity of blood from 8 patients with coronary occlusion at very low rates of shear and without anticoagulation. He described greatly increased viscosity and red cell aggregation, which he defined as the ratio of viscosity at $0.4 \sec^{-1}$ (aggregation effect) to that at $100 \sec^{-1}$ (hematocrit effect). No data were given concerning the stage or severity of the coronary occlusion.

In a subsequent publication (Dintenfass, 1966), further data were presented on 10 patients with acute myocardial infarction, 7 with old myocardial infarctions, and 3 with ischemic heart disease and angina pectoris. The blood viscosity in patients suffering from myocardial infarction and occlusive arterial disease was again much greater than the blood viscosity of normal men and women tested at low rates of shear. Dintenfass (1969) believed that an elevation of viscosity preceded the appearance of clinical symptoms. Our own studies, done with a different technique, have failed to confirm Dintenfass's results. The viscosity of whole blood in balanced oxalate anticoagulant was not increased during acute myocardial infarction. Moreover, no striking alteration of viscosity at low rate of shear was noted. As described in Chapter 2, we have utilized a variety of viscometers to measure shear rate from less than 1 to more than $10^5 \sec^{-1}$ (Charm and Kurland, 1965). The yield stress located by extrapolation to zero shear compared well with values obtained by independent methods. The yield stress in patients with acute myocardial infarction was not different from that in normal persons.

On the other hand, Wells et al. (1969) have shown that red cell aggregation in blood from patients suffering from myocardial infarction was more shear resistant than normal. They reported also the presence of a yield shear stress in pathologic sera not present in blood from normal subjects. It should be noted that studies of the bulbar conjunctiva have revealed striking abnormalities during acute myocardial infarction. Bloch (1955) and Wells (1967) found a highly significant relation between the degree of abnormality in the coronary vessels and in flow patterns in the conjunctival vessels. The relation of blood viscosity and shear rate related alterations in the clotting mechanism (Dintenfass, 1964, 1969) to proneness to thrombosis and to the etiology of myocardial infarction remain uncertain. Both clotting time and platelet adhesiveness have been shown to be shear dependent (Dintenfass, 1969).

The effect of chronic coronary heart disease has been studied in a number of laboratories. Mayer (1964) compared 250 apparently healthy subjects with 86 patients suffering from chronic coronary heart disease. In confirmation of the data of Dintenfass, the patients with coronary disease had higher hematocrit, higher whole blood viscosity, and higher plasma viscosity than the healthy controls. In contrast, Rosenblatt (1965) found no relation between coronary disease and viscosity.

Our own studies undertaken in conjunction with the Framingham heart project are not complete; they suggest, however, that persons for whom there is documented evidence of coronary artery disease have high plasma viscosity but normal whole blood viscosity. Similar results have recently been reported by Isogai et al. (1971). Fukada (1968) found a correlation between serum viscosity and coronary disease.

Elevation of blood viscosity has been noted in other cardiovascular diseases. Eisenberg (1964) studied patients in congestive heart failure and found viscosity to be normal or slightly increased at time of hospital admission; as edema decreased, however, the hematocrit, viscosity, and fibrinogen all rose – probably secondary to a decline in plasma volume relative to red cell mass. Although conclusive studies are not available, it seems likely that the increase in hematocrit and fibrinogen greatly increases the yield stress and the tendency of red cells to agglutinate at low rates of flow. The relation of these changes to a tendency to venous thrombosis during massive diuresis while treating congestive failure is suggestive, but not proven. Eisenberg (1966) has shown increased viscosity within 24 hours in 75% of patients with cerebral thrombosis. There was a pronounced hyperfibrinogenemia, but the correlation of viscosity with fibrinogen was poor.

6.3   ELASTICITY OF RED BLOOD CELLS

The discussion thus far has centered on the role of altered hematocrit in hemodynamics, flow in the microcirculation, and the genesis of vascular disease. In addition to the influence of the volume fraction of red cells, viscosity is also influenced by the elasticity of the red cell and changes in its rigidity or deformability and internal viscosity. In the smallest vessels these factors may be critical. For example, as described in Chapter 2, red cells fixed in acetaldehyde, glutaraldehyde, or formaldehyde are more viscous than normal cells (Chien et al., 1967; Ham et al., 1968; Schmid-Schönbein et al., 1969). Increased shear stress deforms normal erythrocytes and lowers the suspension viscosity but has no effect on the viscosity of hardened cell suspensions.

A clinical counterpart of considerable significance is found in sickle-cell disease. Sickle cells stand between rigid particles and normal red cells (Harris, 1950; Harris et al., 1956). Reduced SS hemoglobin exists in a very viscous form compared with the AA hemoglobin of reduced normal red cells, which permits low internal viscosity (Dintenfass, 1964). When in the sickled form, stroma-free hemoglobin solutions from homozygous sickle disease show extreme increases in viscosity, in resistance to packing, in mechanical fragility, and in difficulty in passing through microfilters that readily permit flow of unsickled forms (Jandl et al., 1961). It has been suggested that sickled cells have lost fluidity and are therefore rigid because of tactoid formation of the hemoglobin. The red cells in sickle-cell trait are less susceptible to the sickling process than those of homozygous disease; even in these cells, however, increased viscosity resulting from hypertonicity may slow flow, permitting deoxygenation and pH reduction to a level critical for sickling (Harris et al., 1956). Violent exercise and high altitude have been precipitants.

Chien et al. (1970) have stressed that the viscosity of HbSS blood exceeds that of normal blood not only during deoxygenation but even under conditions of complete oxygenation. Moreover, both irreversibly sickled cells and non-irreversibly sickled cells possess lower than normal deformability. The altered membrane flexibility and increased internal viscosity may impede capillary flow even in full oxygenation. Under conditions of deoxygenation, aggregation of sickled cells further leads to stasis. The clinical consequences are particularly well seen in the kidney in homozygous sickle-cell disease where thrombosis, papillary necrosis, hematuria, and limited renal function with hyposthenuria have been described (Schlitt and Keitel, 1960; Keitel et al., 1960; Mostofi et al., 1967). Vascular occlusion and infarction have been observed in other beds (Uzsoy, 1964; Kimmelstein, 1948; Schenk, 1964; Finch, 1972).

The clinical severity of various sickle syndromes is related to the rate of increase of viscosity of blood during deoxygenation (Charache and Conley, 1964). The increase of viscosity is determined by the concentration of sickle hemoglobin and by the degree of hemoglobin interaction when more than one type is present. The importance of increased viscosity in the pathogenesis of sickle-cell crises and the demonstration that normal red cells reduce viscosity resulting from conditions of lowered pH and oxygen tension has prompted a prophylactic transfusion program. Anderson et al. (1963) and Levitt et al. (1960) reversed the renal defect in homozygous sickle-cell disease in young children by multiple transfusions. Intravenous urea has been used to break the hydrophobic bonds responsible for sickling (McCurdy and Mahmood, 1971). It has been demonstrated *in vitro* that cyanate shifts the oxygen dissociation curve and inhibits sickling (de Furia et al., 1972).

Hemoglobin C has also been found to be more viscous than normal, leading to decreased deformability and increased blood viscosity (Charache et al., 1967; Murphy, 1968). Significant precipitation of Heinz bodies also makes a cell rigid, probably increases viscosity, and decreases red cell life span (Charache et al., 1967; Murphy, 1968b). Heinz bodies, glutathione–hemoglobin-mixed disulfides, are found in abnormalities of the pentose shunt, unstable hemoglobin syndromes, and thalassemia syndromes. Blood from patients with other types of hemolytic anemia revealed no significant difference in viscosity, regardless of whether the samples were oxygenated or fully reduced (Ham and Castle, 1940). But Schmid-Schönbein and Wells (1969) have been impressed by the red cell membrane hemoglobin abnormality and changes in bulk viscosity in hemolytic anemias and chronic renal and hepatic failure after correction for lowered hematocrit. *In vivo*, the red cell of acquired hemolytic anemias has shown decreased flexibility when traversing capillaries (Guest et al., 1971).

Other properties of red cells also influence viscosity. An increase in hydrogen ion concentration leads to aggregation of red cells, increased internal viscosity, rigidity, and an increase in whole blood viscosity (Dintenfass and Burnard, 1966c).

The rise in viscosity resulting from a decrease in pH may be due partly to changes in size and shape which follow an increase in volume; yet an additional factor is a change in internal viscosity, that is, the red cell membrane or contents or both (Giombi and Burnard, 1970). Hypotonic media increase the yield shear stress of red cells but decrease the viscosity.

Erslev and Atwater (1963) found an exponential relation between the relative viscosity of whole blood and the mean corpuscular hemoglobin concentration. When this measure exceeded 34, viscosity rose sharply. Such values, found mostly in hereditary spherocytosis, may be important for capillary transit and splenic sequestration. Indeed, Murphy (1968a) learned that the small surface in spherocytes influenced the surface-to-volume relationship, especially at low pH, and thus was associated with a less deformable cell and increased viscosity (LaCelle and Weed, 1972).

Relative viscosity of human whole blood is influenced not only by the size of cell but by their shape, as well. The normal biconcave disc shape of the human red cell, with an excess of surface-to-volume, is essential to deformability – a critical property for flow through minute vessels. Decrease in the ratio of surface area to volume by osmotic swelling results in the loss of biconcave shape and lessened flexibility. Although there is a variation in red cell shape in different animal species, the effect of these differences in viscosity is not clear (Stone et al., 1968; Gregerson et al., 1965; Trevan, 1918; Rathe, 1968). In man, a characteristic relation has been noted between whole blood viscosity and relative red cell mass, regardless of the size and number of cells constituting the mass (Strumia and Phillips, 1963). When the red cell count remains constant, however, microcytosis is accompanied by a decrease of relative viscosity of blood and macrocytosis by an increase.

Although intrinsic membrane deformability is significantly related to cellular ATP, calcium, and magnesium and may be affected by pH and pO_2, clinical counterparts are not yet recognized (Weed et al., 1969). The role of such substances may be large in low flow states such as shock, however.

As we have previously discussed (Chapter 2), alterations of other formed elements in the blood have little influence on viscosity. We have found that red cells suspended in platelet-free plasma have the same viscosity as those suspended in normal plasma. Putnam et al. (1965) found no change in viscosity despite platelet variation from 50,000 to $1.9 \times 10^6/cm^3$. It is clear, however, that platelet thromboemboli can have a major influence on blood flow in the microcirculation.

Within normal ranges, the number of white blood cells has no significant influence on viscosity. The viscosity of whole blood in a few cases of acute leukemia has been found to be high, however; perhaps this was because of a high concentration of white blood cells that are more rigid, or perhaps plasma changes were responsible. In our laboratory we have also found white blood cells to be more viscous than an equivalent volume fraction of red blood cells (Steinberg and Charm, 1971).

6.4   PLASMA PROTEINS

Although the major changes in blood viscosity are the result of changes in hematocrit and red cell properties, significant and critical changes also may be produced by alterations in the suspending plasma, particularly at low shear rate. Changes in plasma viscosity have been related to whole blood viscosity at the same hematocrit. Positive correlation of plasma viscosity has been found with total protein, fibrinogen, α_1, α_2, β, and γ globulins; an inverse relation with albumin has been noted (Mayer, 1960; Wells, 1965; Merrill et al., 1965; Somer, 1966). The extent of red cell aggregation and the anomalous rheologic behavior of whole blood have been ascribed to red-cell—fibrinogen interaction (Replogle et al., 1967; Merrill, 1966; Chien, 1967), the extent of the interaction being dependent on each component. Chien et al. have also stressed the importance of serum globulins in shear-dependent aggregation of red cells. In addition, yield shear stress – the force necessary to disrupt the red cell aggregates of motionless blood – is also a function of fibrinogen and globulin concentration (as well as hematocrit) after a minimum concentration has been reached. Yield stress, the major factor in the non-Newtonian property of blood, is particularly relevant at low shear rates; the fraction of total shear represented by yield stress is less significant at high shear rates. The importance of yield stress on microcirculatory flow has not been sufficiently investigated. There are regrettably few clinical studies relating viscosity and yield stress to fibrinogen levels. Merrill et al. (1965) correlated viscosity and fibrinogen content in blood from normal donors but found the relation valid only at fibrinogen concentrations of 210 to 460 mg%. Weaver et al. (1969) found that a raised fibrinogen concentration leads to a greatly increased viscosity at low rates of shear but suggested that the flow reduction from this level might be negligible at the shear rates of a normal circulation. A relevant observation was recorded by Wells (1965) concerning a patient with a major burn; in that case, data were as follows: fibrinogen, 884 mg%; yield stress, 0.21 dyne/cm^2; whole blood hematocrit 48%. In a study of patients with cerebral thrombosis and congestive heart failure, Eisenberg (1964, 1966) noted an increase in viscosity and in plasma fibrinogen concentration in both states but found poor correlation of viscosity to fibrinogen content. The erratic results may be due to inadequate technology for the measurement of circulating fibrinogen. Ditzel (1959) observed that raised plasma fibrinogen was associated with aggregation and sludging of red cells. These findings may be relevant to the increased blood viscosity, increased fibrinogen level, and sludging in conjunctival vessels noted in patients suffering from Raynaud's disease (Pringle, 1965). On the other hand, Begg and Hearns (1966) studied 32 patients, half of whom had vascular disease, and found no significant change in viscosity from variation of plasma fibrinogen between 276 to 1070 mg%. Wayland (1967) described irregularities of the relation of fibrinogen to viscosity and suggested a role for fibrinolytic products (Meiselman et al., 1972). Added fibrinogen *in vivo* produced no effect on rheologic properties of dog's blood between 28 and 560 sec^{-1}.

Other serum proteins are occasionally of marked importance in viscosity, and the physiochemical correlation of structure and viscometric effect is instructive. A hyperviscosity syndrome in macroglobulinemia, originally suggested by Reimann, was described by Fahey (1963, 1965). The clinical manifestations, which included a bleeding diathesis, retinopathy, and visual and neurological disturbances, were associated with elevated serum and blood viscosity. The occurrence of hyperviscosity of the plasma in macroglobulinemia has been frequently confirmed and has been extensively reviewed by Somer (1966). Aggregation of red cells during sedimentation has been described, as well as marked dilatation of all vessels and stagnant flow in conjunctival vessels.

The profound erythrocyte aggregation that has been observed *in vivo* in the pial vessels of macroglobulinemic mice has been related to the magnitude of blood viscosity measured *in vitro* (Rosenblum, 1968). Such data provide a model for understanding the neorologic manifestations of the hyperviscosity syndromes described previously. In more recent work, Rosenblum (1969, 1970) has compared the effects of increased viscosity in macroglobulinemic and poly-cythemic mice. Marked aggregation and vasoconstriction were seen only in macroglobulinemic mice, whereas normal vascular appearance and contractile response were present in polycythemic animals. These interesting discrepancies require us to reconsider the entire relation of the hemodynamic response to increased aggregation, increased yield stress, and increased viscosity; in addition, there is a need to determine the factors that actually impede flow and result in thrombosis.

Similar manifestations of hyperviscosity have been described in multiple myeloma (Kopp, 1967; Somer, 1966; Pruzanski and Watt, 1972; Lindsley et al., 1973) and cryoglobulinemia (Meltzer and Franklin, 1966). Important factors in macroglobulinemia and myeloma are size, protein–protein interaction, and ensuing red cell aggregates. The increase in relative viscosity for a given protein concentration is greater with IgM (mw 1,000,000) than with IgG (mw 160,000) (Fahey, 1965; Barth, 1964). It has been suggested that IgM molecules, which are large and have a high axial–length ratio, have a five-pronged spidery shape emanating from a central ring structure; thus they aggregate and interact rather easily and are unusually susceptible to shear forces. Accordingly, the increase of blood viscosity is greater in macroglobulinemia than in myeloma (Williams, 1968). Occasionally, however, both IgA and IgG myeloma globulins have physical properties that increase viscosity (Benninger and Kreps, 1971). Concentration, temperature-dependent aggregation, and polymerization seem to be important (Pruzanski and Watt, 1972; Lindsley et al., 1973). The prediction of the hemodynamic consequences of macroglobulinemia and myeloma are complicated by the presence of hypervolemia and by a decreased hematocrit (Kopp, 1969). Plasmaphoresis and cyclophosphamide therapy have been demonstrated to be effective in reducing sludge in the conjunctivae vessels and producing subjective improvement both in macroglobulinemia and myeloma (Kopp et al., 1967; Smith et al., 1965).

Increased serum viscosity has been associated with increased concentration of γ globulin and rheumatoid factor in patients with rheumatoid arthritis, systemic lupus erythematosus, and polyarteritis (Cowan and Harkness, 1947; Houstner et al., 1949; Shearn et al., 1963, Isogai, 1971; Jasin et al., 1970). A clinical rheumatoid hyperviscosity syndrome has been described only rarely; in two cases the findings were ascribed to an interaction of rheumatoid factor and intermediate IgG complexes (Jasin et al., 1970).

In view of the importance of microangiopathy and vascular disease in the natural history of diabetes mellitus, viscosity changes are of particular interest. Glucose up to a concentration of 210 mg% and insulin added *in vitro* do not themselves influence viscosity (Gordon, 1969). The decrease in blood viscosity during a glucose tolerance test, shown to be due to hemodilution, is probably not related to the changes in diabetes mellitus. Increased whole blood viscosity, found in 16 nonacidotic long-term diabetic patients, was significantly correlated with α_2 nd β globulin concentrations (Skovborg et al., 1966). Although an increased fibrinogen content of plasma appeared in the diabetic subjects, the concentration of plasma fibrinogen did not correlate with whole blood viscosity – a finding not confirmed by Merrill (1969). Plasma viscosity in the diabetic subjects did not differ from that of the controls, confirming the results of Cogan (1961), although he also failed to note any correlation of viscosity with retinopathy. It was suggested that the blood cells in diabetes behaved abnormally by forming aggregates. These findings are similar to those of Ditzel and Moincet (1959), who recorded increased frequency and extensiveness of red cell aggregation in the conjunctival vessels of young diabetic subjects and even more in those with retinopathy (Ditzel and Skovborg, 1966). These authors, however, reported no alteration of blood viscosity in diabetes of short duration and without retinopathy or nephropathy, in contrast to the recent findings of Isogai (1971). Rees et al. (1968) found no increase in yield stress in diabetic retinopathy without other complications but observed varying degrees of red cell aggregation in the bulbar conjunctiva. When fulminant progressive proliferating retinopathy complicated severe diabetes and renal disease, there was a consistently increased yield stress, along with increased fibrinogen and macroglobulin. In diabetic coma, the change in viscosity may be further accentuated by severe dehydration (Reubi, 1953).

Severe dehydration is also present in nonketotic diabetic coma, in which marked hypertonicity and hyperglycemia are noted, as well. The relative contribution of these derangements to the mortality is not known, but postmortem examination sometimes discloses cerebral infarcts, pelvic venous thrombosis, and pulmonary embolism (Schwartz and Appelbaum, 1968). No studies of viscosity are yet reported in this syndrome, but the rise in hematocrit, the tendency to aggregation described in diabetes, and the marked hypertonicity mentioned earlier will all influence viscosity at low shear rates.

6.5 BLOOD LIPIDS

Because experimental and epidemiologic evidence has linked dietary and circulating fats with the incidence of coronary atherosclerosis and myocardial infarction, the influence of lipids on flow in the microcirculation has been repeatedly considered.

Swank (1951) reported packing and distortion of red blood cells accompanied by some increase in adhesiveness following a large, fat meal. He subsequently noted (Swank, 1954) that viscosity (as reflected by the time for 0.1 ml of blood to flow through a standardized orifice) began to rise about 3 hours after a cream feeding, reached a peak in 6 to 9 hours, and returned to normal by 24 hours. These changes were not due to hematocrit variation. Studies in hamsters showed a 50 to 100% increase in viscosity after a fat meal (Cullen and Swank, 1954). As the chylomicron count began to fall, changes in the stability of the red cell suspension appeared, with increased rouleau formation and increased aggregation. The importance of species difference was indicated when studies in dogs (in contrast to work with hamsters) revealed only a slight equivocal increase in viscosity from fat feeding and, moreover, this change was soon followed by a decrease in blood viscosity (Swank, 1956).

We had studied normal students and could find no change in viscosity of plasma or whole blood 2.5 hours after a fatty meal, whether studied by a capillary viscometer, a cone and plate viscometer at $230 \, \text{sec}^{-1}$, or a coaxial viscometer at a very low shear rate. In fact, in 2 of 52 cases, whole blood viscosity was decreased (Charm et al., 1963). Our observations confirmed those of Shearn and Gousios, 1960) performed following the intravenous infusion of a fat emulsion. Similarly, Watson (1957), who used a Hess viscometer, found only a slight fall in whole blood viscosity after a fat meal with no relation to the degree of lipemia; serum and plasma viscosity were not affected by fat concentration.

On the other hand, a study of 2 hyperlipemic patients by Merrill et al. (1964), revealed that the yield stress reaches a maximum 3 hours after a meal; but this increase did not parallel the rise in triglyceride concentration, which did not reach a maximum for 6 hours and by that time the yield stress was back to normal.

Gelin et al. (1967) found that 4 hypercholesterolemic patients had slightly higher whole blood and plasma viscosity than normal subjects; a fat meal decreased plasma viscosity but increased whole blood viscosity, especially at low rates of shear. Subsequent administration of heparin decreased whole blood viscosity in parallel with the plasma triglyceride level. A review of Gelin's data reveals the changes to be small and inconsistent.

Konttinen and Somer (1963) correlated plasma viscosity and triglycerides in a group of young men at rest and after exercise. In the resting group plasma viscosity did not rise with postprandial triglyceridemia, but after exercise plasma viscosity was elevated in the face of decreased triglycerides.

In population studies, Swank (1962) found that at relatively low lipid intakes the viscosity index was significantly influenced by lipid intake; at higher intakes, however, there was no further effect. Our investigations (Tejada et al., 1964), which compared three socioeconomic groups in Guatemala, revealed no changes in blood viscosity independent of serum total cholesterol and fat intake. Since both these studies were done at high rates of shear, the agglutination effects important at low shear were ignored.

The effect of fatty meals on the visible microcirculation suggests agglutination in some subjects. Williams et al. (1957) found inconsistent agglutination of cells in the bulbar conjunctival circulation in normal students after ingestion of fat; yet there was increased agglutination and plugging of arterioles in a patient 2 weeks after a myocardial infarction. Similar responses were noted by Friedman et al. (1964, 1965), who found marked sludging and capillary ischemia in the conjunctivae of coronary-prone subjects, whereas such effects were rare in others. Duncan et al. (1968) suggested that chlorophenoxy isobutyrate, a hypolipidemic agent, significantly reduces both blood sludging in conjunctival vessels and excessive lipidemia. The relation of the changes in the microcirculation to the decrease in myocardial blood flow and oxygen consumption during postprandial lipemia (Regan et al., 1959, 1961) remains to be clarified.

Striking changes in the microcirculation have been described in a number of important clinical states, but the origin of these changes is probably multifactorial and does not fit readily into the previous classification. Increased blood viscosity has long been recognized in dogs in experimental shock (Seligman et al., 1946). The complex state of the microcirculation in this condition has recently been reviewed (Berman and Fulton, 1965; Shepro and Fulton, 1967). Extensive data are available in animals, and the results vary depending on the individual subject, the species, the site examined, and the type of shock. Low blood pressure, slow flow (decreased rate of shear), alteration of the vascular wall, leukocytosis, platelet thromboembolism, increases in fibrinogen concentration and hematocrit, a change in red cell surface, and a drop in temperature all may influence microcirculatory flow; such conditions tend to increase yield stress and viscosity and to promote aggregation and sludging. Following the drop of blood pressure there is slowing of flow, a decrease in shear rate, and an increase in red blood cell aggregation or rouleau formation and viscosity, particularly in areas of low shear. At this stage, restoration of flow will probably reverse the microcirculatory changes (Branemark, 1967). More prolonged circulatory compromise and stasis lead to further increases in viscosity due to transcapillary fluid shifts, an increase in hematocrit (Chien, 1969), and an increase in the internal viscosity of the red blood cell, which becomes more rigid owing to a decrease in oxygen tension and the development of acidosis (Litwin, 1965; LaCelle and Weed, 1972). Deoxygenation of hemoglobin at reduced pH secondary to an increase in pCO_2 or metabolites causes sphering and rigidity of the cell, which in turn increases viscosity, reduces velocity, and sets up a vicious cycle.

Although the influence of rheologic changes on flow in small arterioles and capillaries is most often emphasized, consideration should also be given to the influence of such changes on the postcapillary venous system. Here, where shear stresses are low, viscous resistance due to increased hematocrit, acidosis, or hypoxia may be particularly important. Since shock is often associated with an acute disease process, there is further tendency for red cells to adhere, resisting disaggregation. When in addition to reduced flow rates there is tissue damage, wall adherence of red cells, white cells, and platelets impedes flow; in addition, microemboli and mixed microthrombi of fibrin, platelets, red cells, and white cells produce microvascular obstruction and additional stasis, hypoxia, and acidosis. At the irreversible stage of shock, effective tissue perfusion may be further restricted by damage to the endothelial lining of small vessels and capillaries with fibrin deposition and small thrombi, an element of intravascular coagulation, extensive vasospasm, and the opening of AV shunts (Renkin, 1968; West, 1969).

Alteration of microvascular flow has been reported following incompatible blood transfusion, malarial crises (Knisely, 1965), and anaphylaxis (Irwin, 1964). Intravascular aggregation has been described following a variety of tissue trauma such as fracture, contusion, burns, cold, surgery (Gelin, 1959, 1961), myocardial infarction (Bloch, 1955), acute alcoholism (Lee, 1966), bacterial pneumonia, and poliomyelitis. The pathogenesis of aggregation and increased viscosity in these states has not been completely characterized. Consideration has been given to alteration of intercellular changes and changes in plasma proteins and the red cell surface. An increase in plasma viscosity has been found (Gelin, 1961); striking increases in fibrinogen levels are sometimes observed (Wells, 1965; Isogai, 1971). A body of evidence suggests the presence of an abnormal coating on the red cell in trauma and disease (Bloch, 1956; Knisely,

1965; Lee, 1968). Shear-rate-resistant red cell aggregation has been noted following surgical trauma (Wells et al., 1968). Whatever the cause of the initial aggregation, its consequences include red cell sequestration and destruction, as well as the "anemia of injury" (Gelin, 1956). Once the aggregates have formed, the potential exists for secondary hemodynamic effects of the type described earlier in shock. No increase in viscosity was found in the absence of shock in combat casualties, however (McNamara et al., 1972).

Equally complex are the changes observed during prolonged extracorporeal circulation. Erythrocyte aggregation, which has been seen both in dog and man (Long et al., 1961), has been cited as one of the causes of postpump anemia and a rise in plasma hemoglobin (De Wall et al., 1959). On the other hand, substantial hemodilution with plasma expanders results in a decrease in whole blood viscosity. Moreover, these changes are complicated by the frequent presence of hypothermia. Reduction of temperature increases viscosity and yield stress (see Chapter 2; Rand et al., 1964; Virgilio et al., 1964), at least when the hematocrit value exceeds 50% (Marty et al., 1971). Lowering the temperature is said to increase aggregation in experimental animals (Gelin and Lofstrom, 1955; Bigelow et al., 1950). These changes result in part from the hemoconcentration of cooling (Eiseman and Spencer, 1962). Such a tendency would be abetted by any associated low flow, metabolic acidosis, or hypoxia. The importance of these factors has been demonstrated by Keen and Gerbode (1963), who showed that intravascular agglutination of erythrocytes in hypothermic dogs could be prevented by adequate maintenance of blood pressure. They ascribed the agglutination to poor capillary perfusion and circulatory failure rather than temperature. These changes must be viewed against the background of seriously ill patients with cardiac disease with high preoperative blood viscosity and large postoperative increase in viscosity (Barnett and Meilman, 1972).

In view of the extensive hemodynamic and metabolic consequences that have been ascribed to intravascular erythrocyte aggregation, it is natural that efforts should have been made to improve the suspension stability of whole blood. Fajers and Gelin (1959) noted that low molecular weight dextran (LMD) was capable of reducing the red cell loss associated with injury. Improvement of aggregation resulting from high molecular weight dextran, shock, or extra-corporeal circulation was reported to result from administration of LMD. A flood of observations attested to the clinical success of this agent. However, there remains considerable dispute regarding the mechanism of its reputed therapeutic usefulness. Some theorize that LMD improves or increases red cell negativity. Others assert that its action appears to result from alteration of the surface material of red cells, reducing bonding forces (Lee, 1968). However, a large body of evidence suggests that the action of dextran results from the significant hemodilution it produces (Wells, 1968; Meiselman and Merrill, 1968; Replogle et al., 1965, 1967). In the studies cited, when hemodilution was avoided by infusing LMD in a suspension of packed red blood cells, keeping the hematocrit constant, no effect on blood flow during hemorrhagic hypotension was observed. Similarly, *in vitro* studies by Meiselman et al. (1967) revealed no decrease in viscosity or yield stress when dextran was added to whole blood, provided the hematocrit was kept constant. As in other studies, the problem of species differences was important; for example, Engeset et al. (1967) used an *in vitro* test of aggregation and found Dextran 40 to have a specific dispersing effect on aggregated human or canine cells but not on rabbit cells. The conflict is not yet resolved between those ascribing a specific disaggregating effect to LMD and those who feel that its effect is to reduce viscosity by hemodilution (Derrick and Guest, 1971).

6.6   SUMMARY

Changes in viscosity and yield stress play a significant role in clinical medicine. An increased incidence of occlusive vascular disease has been demonstrated in a number of conditions characterized by increased viscosity. The rise in viscosity can result from increased hematocrit (as in polycythemia), increased rigidity of cells (as in homozygous sickle-cell disease), or altered plasma proteins (as in macroglobulinemia). In addition, increased aggregation has been associated with a variety of tissue injuries, but the mechanism of this aggregation remains the subject of speculation. In some cases it is apparently related to fibrinogen, in some to other plasma proteins, and in others possibly to altered properties of the red cell surface. A tendency to hyperviscosity or aggregation is potentiated by the occurrence of acidosis or by a drop of cardiac output, velocity of blood flow, perfusion pressure, or temperature. The entire picture may be further accentuated by vascular reactions. An increasing number of therapeutic interventions have demonstrated their clinically usefulness.

Condition	Clinical Approach
Polycythemia	Remove cause (e.g., tumor)
	Venesection
	Prevent dehydration
	Partial exchange transfusion,
	Dilution
Dysproteinemia	
Macroglobulinemia	Exchange transfusion
Myeloma	Cyclophosphamide
Enhanced aggregation	Disaggregation: ? dextran
	Dilution: water, dextran, albumin
	Improve cardiac status
	Prevent acidosis

References

Abbrecht, P. H. (1968). "An outline of renal structure and function." *Chem. Eng. Prog. Symp. Ser.* 84 (64), p. 1.

Adams, T. and P. F. Iampietro (1968). "Temperature regulation." In *"Exercise Physiology"*, H. B. Falls (Ed.). Academic Press, New York, p. 173.

Aetland, P. and B. Highman (1971). "Effects of polycythemia and altitude hypoxia on rat heart and exercise tolerance." *Am. J. Physiol.* 221 (2), p. 228.

Alvarez, O. A. and D. L. Yudlevich (1969). "Heat capillary permeability to lipid insoluble molecules." *J. Physiol. (London)* 202, p. 45.

Ambrose, E. J. (1965). *Cell Electrophoresis.* Little, Brown, Boston, p. 178.

Anderson, R., M. Cassell, and H. Chaplin, Jr. (1963). "Effect of normal cells on viscosity of sickle-cell blood." *Arch. Int. Med.* 3, p. 286.

Aroesty, J. and J. F. Gross, (1970). "Convection and diffusion in the microcirculation." *Microvasc. Res.* 2, p. 247.

Baez, S. (1968). "Vascular smooth muscle: quantification of cell thickness in the walls of arterioles in the living animal in situ." *Science* 159, p. 536.

Balke, B. (1964). "Cardiac performance in relation to altitude." *Am. J. Cardiol.* 14, p. 796.

Barbee, J. H. and G. R. Cokelet (1971). "The Fahraeus effect." *Microvasc. Res.* 3, p. 6.

Barbee, J. H. and G. R. Cokelet (1971). "Prediction of blood flow in tubes with diameters as small as 29." *Microvasc. Res.* 3, p. 17.

Barbee, J. H. and G. R. Cokelet (1972). "The flow of human blood through small capillary tubes." Abstracted in *Microvasc. Res.* 4, p. 320.

Barbee, J. H. (1973). "Effect of temperature on blood viscosity." *Biorheology* 10, p. 1.

Barnet, B. and E. Meilman (1972). "Measurement of the rheological properties of biological fluids. III. Viscoelastic properties of blood serum." *Biorheology* 9, p.2, 265.

Barth, W. F. (1964). "Viscosimetry in serum in relation to serum globulins." In *Serum Proteins and the Dipproteinemias*, I. W. Sunderman and F. W. Sunderman (Eds.). Lippincott, Philadelphia, Chapter 12.

Basler, A. (1918). Über die Blutbewegung in den Kapillaren. I. Mitteilung Registriering der Stromungsgeschwindigkeit." *Pflugers Arch Ges. Physiol.* 171, p. 134.

Baum, R. S. (1967). "Hyperviscous blood and perinatal pathology." Abstracted in *Pediatr. Res.* 1, p. 288.

Baum, R. (1966). "Viscous forces in neonatal polycythemia." Abstracted in *Pediatrics* 69, p. 975.

Bayliss, L. E. (1952). In *Rheology of Blood and Lymph. Deformation and Flow in Biological Systems,* A. Frey-Wyssling (Ed.). Interscience, New York., p. 354.

Bayliss, L. E. (1959). "The axial drift of red cells when blood flows in a narrow tube." *J. Physiol.* 149, p. 593.

Bayliss, L. E. (1960). "The anomalous viscosity of blood." In *Flow Properties of Blood*, A. L. Copley and G. Stainsby (Eds.). Pergamon Press, New York, p. 290

Begg, T. B. and J. B. Hearns (1966). "Components in blood viscosity." *Clin. Sci.* 31, p. 87.

Benis, A. M., S. Usami and S. Chien (1970). "Effect of hematocrit and inertial losses on pressure–flow relations in the isolated hind paw of the dog." *Circ. Res.* 27, p. 1047.

Benis, A. M. and J. Lacoste (1968a). "Study of erythrocyte aggregation by blood viscometry at low shear rates using a balance method." *Circ. Res.* 22, p. 29.

Benis, A. M. and J. Lacoste (1968b). "Distribution of blood flow in vascular beds: Model study of geometrical and hydrodynamical effects." *Biorheology* 5, p. 147.

Benis, A., S. Usami and S. Chien (1971). "Determination of the shear stress–shear rate relation for blood by Couette viscometry." *Biorheology* 8, p. 65.

Bennet, L. (1967). "Red cell slip at a wall *in vitro*." *Science* 155, p. 1554.

Benninger, G. W. and S. I. Kreps (1971). "Agregation phenomenon in an IgG multiple myeloma resulting in the hyperviscosity syndrome." *Am. J. Med.* 51, p. 287.

Bergentz, S. E., L. E. Gelin, S. E. Lindell and C. M. Rudenstay (1965). "The effect of trauma on equilibrium of C_r^{15} tagged red cells." In *3rd European Conference on Microcirculation, Jerusalem 1964*, Vol. 7. Karger, New York, p. 242.

Berman, H. J., E. W. Merrill and W. G. Margetts (1964). "Effect of dextrans on the rheological properties of hamster blood." *Physiologist* 7, p. 88.

Berman, H. J. (1965). "Rheological properties of the microvasculature." *Bibl. Anat.* 7, p. 29.

Berman, H. J. and G. P. Fulton (1965). "The microcirculation as related to shock." In *Shock and Hypotensions*, Lewis C. Mills and J. H. Moyer (Eds.). Grune & Stratton, New York, p. 198.

Berman, H. J. and R. L. Fuhro (1969). Effect of rate of shear on the shape of the velocity profile and orientation of red cells in arterioles." *Bibl. Anat.* 10, p. 32; Karger, Basel, New York.

Berman, H. J. and R. L. Fuhror (1966). Personal communication.

Berne, M. R. and M. N. Levy (1972). In *Cardiovascular Physiology* Mosby, St. Louis, Mo., p. 107.

Bigelow, W. G., R. O. Heimbecker, and R. C. Harrison (1949). "Intravascular agglutination (sludged blood). Vascular stasis and sedimentation rate of blood in trauma." *Arch. Surg.* 59, p. 667.

Bingham, E. C. and G. F. White (1911). *J. Am. Chem. Soc.* 23, p. 1257. Cited from Bayliss (1962).

Blackshear, P. L., Jr., F. D. Dorman, M. S. Gupta, K. Kilrara (1969). "Particle motion in flowing blood." *Delivered at 2nd International Conference on Hemorheology*, Heidelberg, Germany.

Block, E. H. (1955). "*In vivo* microscopic observations of circulating blood in acute myocardial infarction." *Am. J. Med. Sci.* 229, p. 280

Bloch, E. H., A. Powell, H. T. Merryman, L. Warner, and E. Kafig (1956). "A comparison of the surfaces of human erythrocytes from health and disease by *in vivo* light microscopy and *in vitro* electronmicroscopy." *Angiology* 7, p. 489.

Bloch, E. H., R. S. McGuskey, G. Tucker, and J. Menan (1961). "The effect of cellular aggregation as pressure–flow relationships on the microvascular system." *Angiology* 12, p. 473.

Bloch, E. H. (1962). "A quantitative study of hemodynamics in the living microvascular systems." *Am. J. Anat.* 110 (2), p. 125.

Bloch, E. H. (1965). "Some principles of hemodynamics in the microvascular system." In *Shock and Hypotension*, Lewis C. Mills and J. H. Moyer (Eds.). Grune & Stratton, New York, p. 194.

Blum, J. J. (1960). "Concentration profiles in and around capillaries." *Am. J. Physiol.* 198, p. 991.

Boardman, G. and R. L. Whitmore (1961). "Static measurement of yield stress." *Lab. Pract.* 10, p. 782.

Brandt, A. and G. Bugliarello (1965). "A simplified model of the flow in the plasmatic gaps of the smaller circulatory vessels." *Proc. 18th ACEMB*, Philadelphia.

Branemark, P. I. and H. Harders (1963). "Intravital analysis of microvascular form and function in man." *Lancet* 2, p. 1197.

Branemark, P. J. (1968). "Rheologic aspects of low flow states." In *Microcirculation as Related to Shock*, D. Shepro and G. P. Fulton (Eds.). Academic Press, New York, p. 161.

Brooks, D. E., J. W. Goodwin, and G. V. F. Seaman (1970). "Interactions among erythrocytes under shear." *J. Appl. Physiol.* 28 (2), p. 172.

Brooks, D. E. and G. V. F. Seaman (1971). "Role of mutual cellular repulsions in the rheology of concentrated red blood cell suspensions." In *Theoretical and Clinical Hemorheology*, H. Hartet and A. L. Copley (Eds.), (1971), p. 127.

Brooks, G. and G. V. F. Seaman (1972). "An electroviscous effect in the erythrocytes suspensions." First International Conference of Biorheology, Lyon, France, September 1972.

Brown, G. G. (1960). In *Unit Operations*. Wiley, New York, p. 131.

Brown, S. M., H. S. Gilbert, S. Krauss, and L. R. Wasserman (1971). "Spurious (relative) polycythemia: A nonexistent disease." *Am. J. Med.* 50, p. 200.

Bugliarello, G. and G. C. Hsiao (1964). "Phase separations in suspensions flowing through bifurications: A simplified hemodynamic model." *Science* 143, p. 469.

Bugliarello, G. and E. D. Jackson (1964). "Random walk study of convective diffusion." *J. Eng. Mech. Div. Proc. Am. Soc. Civ. Eng.*, p. 49.

Bugliarello, G., C. Kapur, and G. Hsiao (1965). "The profile viscosity and other characteristics of blood flow in a non-uniform shear field." *Symposium on Biorheology*, A. L. Copley (Ed.), (1965), p. 351.

Bugliarello, G. and J. W. Hoskins (1966). "Stochiastic simulation of convective diffusion in the axial plasmatic gaps of capillaries." *Proceedings of the 19th Annual Conference on Engineering in Medicine and Biology, San Fransisco.*

Bugliarello, G., T. K. Hung, and C. E. James, Jr. (1971a). "Model studies of hydrodynamic characteristics of an erythrocyte. III. Drag in an erythrocyte–erythrocyte interaction." In *Theoretical and Clinical Hemorheology*, H. Hartert and A. L. Copley (Eds.)., (1971), p. 30.

Bugliarello, G., T. K. Hung, and M. H. Weissman (1971b). "A numerical model for oscillatory flow and oxygen transfer in the axial plasmatic gaps of capillaries. 1. Two-dimensional disklike rigid erythrocytes." In *Theoretical and Clinical Hemorheology*, H. Hartert and A. L. Copley (Eds.)., (1971), p. 60.

Bugliarello, G. and G. C. Hsiao (1970). "A mathematical model of the flow in the axial plasmatic gaps of the smaller vessels." *Biorheology*, 7, p. 5.

Bugliarello, G. and J. Sevilla, (1970). "Velocity distribution and other characteristics of steady and pulsatile flow in fine glass tubes." *Biorheology* 7 (2), p. 85.

Burch, G. E. and N. P. DePasquale (1961). "Erythrocytosis and ischemic myocardial disease." *Am. Heart J.* 62, p. 139.

Burch, G. E. and N. P. DePasquale (1962). "The hematocrit in patients with myocardial infarction." *JAMA* 180, p. 63.

Burch, G. E. and N. P. DePasquale (1963). "Phlebotomy – Use in patients with erythrocytosis and ischemic heart disease." *Arch. Int. Med.* 3, p. 687.

Burch, G. E. and N. P. DePasquale (1965). "Hematocrit, viscosity and coronary blood flow." *Dis. Chest* 48, p. 225.

Burris, M. D. and W. R. Arrowsmith (1953). "Vascular complications of polycythemia vera." *Surg. Clin.* 33, p. 1023.

Burton, A. C. (1965). *Physiology and Biophysics of the Circulation.* Year Book, Medical Publishers, Chicago.

Burton, A. C. (1954). "Relation of structure to function of tissues of the walls of blood vessels." *Physiol. Rev.* 34, p. 619.

Butler, J. A. V. (1951). *Electrical Phenomena at Interphases.* Macmillan, New York.

Calabresi, P. and O. O. Meyer (1959). "Polycythemia vera. 1. Clinical and laboratory manifestations." *Am. Int. Med.* 50, p. 1182.

Case, R. B., E. Berglund and S. J. Sarnoff (1955). "Ventricular function. VII. Changes in coronary resistance and ventricular function resulting from acutely induced anemia and the effect thereon of coronary stenosis." *Am. J. Med.* 18, p. 397.

Casson, N. (1958). "A flow equation for pigment—oil suspensions of the printing ink type." In *Rheology of Disperse Systems*, C. C. Mill (Ed.), Pergamon Press, New York. p. 84.

Castaneda, A. R., E. F. Bernstein, and R. L. Varco (1965). "The effect of polyvinylprotedone, mannitol, dextrose and of various dextrans on red cell charge." *3rd European Conference on Microcirculation, Jerusalem, 1964, Bibl. Anat.* 7, p. 262.

Castle, W. B. and J. H. Jandl (1966). "Blood viscosity and blood volume: Opposing influences upon oxygen transport in polychthemia." *Sem. Hematol.* 3, 193.

Cerny, L, C., F. B. Cook, and C. C. Walker (1962). "Rheology of blood." *Am. J. Physiol.* 202 (6), p. 1188.

Cerny, L. C. and W. P. Walawender (1966). "Blood flow in rigid tubes." *Am. J. Physiol.* 210 (2), p. 341.

Cerny, L. C., J. D. Grauz, and H. James (1968). "The effectiveness of plasma expanders, an osmotic pressure and viscosity study." *Biorheology* 5 (2), p. 103.

Chang, C. C. and H. B. Atabek (1961). "The inlet length for oscillatory flow and its effects on the determination of the rate of flow in arteries." *Phys. Med. Biol.* 6, p. 303.

Charache, S. and C. L. Conley (1964). "Rate of sickling of red cells during deoxygenation of blood from persons with various sickling disorders." *Blood* 24, p. 25.

Charache, S., C. L. Conley, D. F. Waugh, R. J. Ugoretz, and J. R. Spurrell (1967). "Pathogenesis of hemolytic anemia in homozygous hemoglobin C disease." *J. Clin. Invest.* 46, p. 1795.

Charm, S. E. and G. S. Kurland (1962). "The flow behaviour and shear stress—shear rate characteristics of canine blood." *Am. J. Physiol.* 203 (3), p. 417.

Charm, S. E., W. McComis, C. Tejada, and G. Kurland (1963). "Effect of a fatty meal on whole blood and plasma viscosity." *J. Appl. Physiol.* 18 (6), p. 1217.

Charm, S. E., W. McComis, and G. S. Kurland (1964). "Rheology and structure of blood suspensions." *J. Appl. Physiol.* 19 (1) p. 127.

Charm, S. E. and G. S. Kurland (1965a). "Viscometry of human blood for shear rates of $0-100,000 \text{ sec}^{-1}$." *Nature* 206 (4984), p. 617.

Charm, S. E., G. S. Kurland, W. McComis, and C. Song (1965b). "Energy losses in steady and pulsatile blood flow." *3rd European Conference on Microcirculation, Jerusalem, 1964. Bibl. Anat.* 17, p. 340.

Charm, S. E. and G. S. Kurland (1966a). "On the significance of the Reynolds number in blood flow." *Biorheology* 3, p. 163.

Charm, S. E. and F. Nelson (1967). Flow and deformation of red cells in capillaries." *4th European Conference on Microcirculation, Cambridge, England. Bibl. Anat.* 9, p. 246.

Charm, S. E. and G. S. Kurland (1967a). "Static method for determining blood yield stress." *Nature* 216 (5120), p. 1121.

Charm, S. E. and G. S. Kurland (1967b). "Blood flow in non-uniform tapered capillary tubes." *Biorheology*, 4, p. 175.

Charm, S. E., G. S. Kurland, and S. Brown (1968a). "The influence of radial distribution and marginal plasma layer on the flow of red cell suspensions." *Biorheology* 5, p. 15.

Charm, S. E., S. Brown, and G. S. Kurland (1968). "On the characteristics of the marginal plasma layer." In *Hemorheology*, A. L. Copley (Ed.), (1968), p. 403.

Charm, S. E., B. Paltiel, and G. S. Kurland (1968b). "Heat transfer coefficients in blood flow." *Biorheology* 5, p. 133.

Charm, S. E., J. M. Moran, and G. S. Kurland (1968c). Unpublished studies on plasma viscosity and atherosclerosis.

Charm, S. E., G. S. Kurland, and M. S. Schwartz (1969a). "Absence of a transition in the viscosity of human blood between shear rates of $20-100$ sec^{-1}." *J. Appl. Physiol.* 26 (3), p. 389.

Charm, S. E. and G. S. Kurland (1969b). "The discrepancy in measuring blood in Couette, cone and plate, and capillary tube viscometers." *J. Appl. Physiol.* 25 (6), p. 786.

Charm, S. E. and G. S. Kurland (1969c). "Temperature effects on blood viscosity." Unpublished data.

Charm, S. E. and B. L. Wong (1970). "Shear degradation of fibrinogen in the circulation." *Science* 170, p. 466.

Chien, S. (1969). "Blood rheology and its relation to flow resistance and transcapillary exchange with surgical reference to shock." *Adv. Microcirc.* 2, p. 89.

Chien, S., S. Usami, and J. F. Bertles (1970). "Abnormal rheology of oxygenated blood in sickle-cell anemia." *J. Clin. Invest.* 49, p. 623.

Chien, S., S. Usami, H. Taylor, J. S. Liniberg, and M. Gregerson (1966). "The effects of hematocrit and plasma protein on human blood rheology at low shear rates." *J. Appl. Physiol.* 21 (1), p. 81.

Chien, S., S. Usami, and R. Dellenback (1967). "Blood viscosity: Influence of erythrocyte deformation." *Science* 157, p. 827.

Chien, S., R. J. Dellenback, S. Usami, G. Seaman, and M. Gregersen (1968). "Centrifugal packing of suspensions of erythrocytes hardened with acetaldehyde." *Proc. Soc. Exp. Biol. Med.* 127, p. 982.

Chien, S., S. Usami, R. J. Dellenback, C. A. Bryant, and M. Gregersen (1971a). "Change of erythrocyte deformability during fixation in acetaldehyde." In *Theoretical and Clinical Hemorheology*, H. Hartert and A. L. Copley (Eds.)., (1971), p. 136.

Chien, S., S. Usami, R. J. Dellenback, and M. Gregersen (1971b). "Influence of fibrinogen and globulins on blood rheology at low shear rates: Comparison among elephant, dog and man." In *Theoretical and Clinical Hemorheology*, H. Hartert and A. L. Copley, (Eds.)., (1971), p. 136.

Chien, S., S. Usami, R. J. Dellenback, and M. I. Gregersen (1970). "Shear dependent deformation of erythrocytes in rheology of human blood." *Am. J. Physiol.* 219, p. 136.

Chien, S., S. Usami, and A Rowe (1971). "Rheological properties of red cells stored in liquid N_2." *J. Lab. Clin. Med.* 78 (1), p. 175.

Chievits, E. and T. Thiede (1962). "Complications and courses of death in polycythemia vera." *Acta Med.* 171, p. 513.

Clementi, F. and G. E. Palade (1969). "Intestinal capillaries. II. Structural effects of EDTA and histamine." *J. Cell Biol.* 42, p. 706.

Cobb, L. A., R. J. Kramer, and C. A. Finch (1960). "Circulatory effects of chronic hypervolemia in polycythemia vera." 39, p. 1722.

Cogan, G., L. Merola, and P. R. Laibson (1961). "Blood viscosity, serum hexosamine and diabetic retinopathy." *Diabetes* 10, p. 393.

Cokelet, G. R. (1963a). "The rheology of human blood." *Doctoral disertation*, M.I.T., Cambridge, Mass.

Cokelet, G. R., E. W. Merrill, E. R. Gilliland, H.Shin, A. Britten, and R. E. Wells (1963b). "Rheology of human blood: Measurement near and at zero shear rate." *Trans. Soc. Rheol.* 7, p. 303.

Cokelet, G. R. (1967). "Comments on the Fahraeus-Lindquist effect." *Biorheology* 4 (3), p. 123.

Cokelet, G. R. and H. J. Meiselman (1968). "Rheological comparison of hemoglobin solutions and erythrocyte suspensions." *Science* 162, p. 276.

Collin, H. B. (1969). "Ultrastructure of fenestrated blood capillaries in extra-ocular muscles" *Exp. Eye Res.* 8, p. 16.

Conley, C. L., R. P. Russell, C. B. Thomas, and P. A. Tumultz (1964). "Hematocrit values in coronary artery disease." *Arch. Int. Med.* 113, p. 170.

Copley, A. L. (1960). In *Flow properties of Blood and Other Biological Fluids*, A. L. Copley, and G. Stainsby (Eds.). Pergamon Press, New York, p. 97.

Copley, A. L. (1953). *Abstracts of Communications* , 19th International Physiological Congress, Montreal, Canada, p. 280.

Copley, A. L. and G. W. Scott-Blair (1960). In *Flow properties of Blood and Other Biological Suspensions*, A. L. Copley and G. Stainsby (Eds.). Pergamon Press, New York, p. 117.

Copley, A. L. (Ed.) (1965). *Symposium on Biorheology: Proceedings of the Fourth International Conference on Rheology*. Interscience, New York.

Copley, A. L., B. W. Luchini, and E. W. Whelan (1967). "On the rate of fibrinogen–fibrin complexes in erythrocyte aggregation and flow properties of blood." *Biorheology* 4, p. 87.

Copley, A. L. (Ed.) (1968). *Hemorheology: Proceedings of the First International Conference on Hemorheology, University of Iceland, Beykjavik, 1966*. Pergamon Press, New York.

Copley, A. (1971). Non-Newtonian behavior of surface layers of human plasma protein systems and a new concept of the initiation of thrombosis. *Biorheology* 8 p. 79.

Copley, A. and R. King (1972). "The action of human red cells and platelets on viscous resistance of plasma protein systems." First International Conference of Biorheology, Lyon, France, September 1972.

Copley. A. L., C. R. Huang, and R. G. King (1973). "Rheogoniometer studies of whole human blood at shear rates from 1000 to 0.0009 sec⁻¹. Part I. Experimental findings." *Biorheology* 10, p. 17.

Coulter, N. A., Jr. and J. R. Pappenheimer (1949). "Turbulence in flowing blood." *Am. J. Physiol.* 159, p. 401.

Cowan, I. C. and J. Harkness (1947). "Plasma viscosity in rheumatic diseases." *Brit. Med. J.* 2, p. 686.

Crowell, J. W. and E. E. Smith (1967). "Determinant of the optimal hematocrit." *J. Appl. Physiol.* **22**, p. 501.

Cullen, C. F. and R. L. Swank (1954). "Intravascular aggregation and adhesiveness of the blood elements associated with plimentary hipenia and injections of large molecular substances." *Circulation* **9**, p. 335.

Danks, D. M. and L. H. Stevens (1964). "Neonatal respiratory distress associated with a high hematocrit reading." *Lancet* **2**, p. 499.

Danon, D., Y. Marikovsky, and E. Skutelsky (1971). "The sequestration of old erythrocytes and expulsed nuclei from the circulation of mammalians." Delivered at 2nd International Conference on Hemorheology, Heidelberg, Germany.

Davis, R. E. and H. J. Woodliff (1966). "Plasma viscosity and the erythrocyte sedimentation rate." *Med. J. Aust.* **2**, p. 265.

Dawber, T. R. and W. B. Kannel (1961). "Susceptibility to coronary heart disease." *Mod. Conc. Cardiovasc. Dis.* **30**, p. 671.

Defares, J. G., J. J. Osborn, and H. Hara (1963). "Theoretical synthesis of the cardiovascular system. Study I: The controlled system." *Acta Physiol. Pharmacol.* **12**, p. 189.

de Furia, F. G., D. R. Miller, A. Cerami, and J, M. Manning (1972). "The effects of cyanate in vitro on red blood cell metabolism and function in sickle cell anemia." *J. Clin. Invest.* **51**, p.566.

Den Hartog, J. P. (1952). In *Advanced Strength of Materials.* McGraw-Hill, New York, p. 119.

DePasquale, N. P. and G. E. Burch (1963). "Hematocrit in women with myocardial infarction." *JAMA* **183**, p. 142.

Dhall, D. P., J. Engeset, F. N. McKenzie, and N. A. Matheson (1969). "Screen filtration of blood – An evaluation." *Cardiovasc. Res.* **3**, p. 147.

DeWall, R. A., D. M. Long, S. J. Gernmill, and C. W. Hilleher (1959). "Certain blood changes in patients undergoing extracorporeal circulation." *J. Thorac. Surg.* **37**, p. 325.

Dick, D. A. T. (1966). In *Cell Water.* Butterworths, Washington, D.C. p. 64.

Dintenfass, L. (1963a). "An application of a cone-in-cone viscometer to the study of viscosity, thixotropy and clotting of blood." *Biorheology* **2**, p. 91.

Dintenfass, L. (1963b). "Blood rheology in cardio-vascular disease." *Nature* **199**, p. 813.

Dintenfass, L. (1964a). "Rheology of packed red blood cell containing hemoglobins A-A-S-A and S-S." *J. Lab. Clin. Med.* **64** (41), p. 594.

Dintenfass, L. (1964b). "Viscosity and clotting of blood in venous thrombosis and coronary occlusion." *Circ. Res.* **14**, p. 1.

Dintenfass, L. (1965). "Some observations on the viscosity of pathological human blood plasma." *Throm Diathesis Haemorrh.* **13** (3/4) p. 492.

Dintenfass, L., D. G. Julian, and G. E. Miller (1966a). "Viscosity of blood in normal subjects and in patients suffering from coronary occlusion and arterial thrombosis." *Am. Heart J.* **71**, p. 587.

Dintenfass, L. (1966b). "A preliminary outline of the blood high viscosity syndromes." *Arch. Int. Med.* **18**, p. 427.

Dintenfass, L. and E. D. Burnard (1966c). "Effect of hydrogen on the *in vitro* viscosity of packed red cells and blood at high hematocrits." *Med. J. Aust.* **1**, p. 1072.

Dintenfass, L. (1968a). "Internal viscosity of the red cell and a blood viscosity equation." *Nature* **219** (5757), p. 956.

218 References

Dintenfass, L. (1968b). "Blood viscosity internal fluidity of the red cell, dynamic coagulation and the critical capillary radius as factors in physiology and pathology of circulation and microcirculation." *Med. J. Aust.* 1, p. 688.

Dintenfass, L. (1969). "Blood rheology in pathogenesis of the coronary heart diseases." *Am. Heart J.* 77, p. 139.

Dintenfass, L. (1971). "Considerations of the internal viscosity of the red cell and of the rheology of the red cell membrane and of the effects of these factors on blood flow." In *Theoretical and Clinical Hemorheology*, H. Hartert and A. L. Copley, (Eds.)., (1971), p. 174.

Dintenfass, L. (1971). *Blood Microrheology: Viscosity Factors in Blood Flow, Ischalmia and Thrombosis.* Appleton-Century-Crofts, New York.

Ditzel, J. and P. Moincet (1959a). "Changes in serum protein, lipoproteins and protein-bound carbohydrates in relation to pathologic alterations in the microcirculation of diabetic subject." *J. Lab. Clin. Med.* 54, p. 843.

Ditzel, J. (1959b). "Relationship of blood protein composition to intravascular erythrocyte aggregation (sludged blood)." *Acta Med. Scand.* 164, Suppl. B43.

Ditzel, J. and F. Skovborg (1968). "Hemorheological investigations in relation to diabetes mellitus and its angiopathy." *Hemorheology*, Pergamon Press, New York, p. 751.

Ditzel, J., H. O. Bang, and N. Thorsen (1968). "Myocardial infarction and whole-blood viscosity." *Acta Med. Scand.* 183, p. 577.

Dix, F. S., and G. W. Scott-Blair (1940). "On the flow of suspensions through narrow tubes." *J. Appl. Phys.* 2, p. 575.

Djojosugito, A. M., B. Folkow, B. Oberg, and S. White (1970). "A comparison of blood viscosity measured in vitro and in a vascular bed." *Acta Physiol. Scand.* 78, pp. 70–84.

Dow, P., F. P. Hahn, and W. F. Hamilton (1946). "Simultaneous transport of T-1824 and radioactive red cells through the heart and lungs." *Am. J. Physiol.* 147, p. 493.

Dow, P. and W. F. Hamilton (1939). "An experimental study of the velocity of the pulse wave through the aorta." *Am. J. Physiol.* 125, p. 60.

Duling, B. R. and R. M. Berne (1970). "Longitudinal gradients in periarteriolar oxygen tension: Possible mechanism for the participation of oxygen in local regulation of blood flow." *Circ. Res.* 27, p. 669.

Duncan, G. G., F. A. Elliott, T. G. Duncan and J. Schatanoff (1968). "Some clinical potentials of chlorophenoxyisobutirete (clofibrate) therapy." *Metabolism* 17, p. 457.

duPre Denning, A. and J. Watson (1900). From "The emergence of rheology by Hershel Markovitz." *Phys. Today* 21 (4), p. 23, April 1968.

Eckstein, R. W. (1955). "Development of interarterial anastomoses by chronic anemia." *Circ. Res.* 3, p. 306.

Ehrly, A. M. (1968). "Reduction in blood viscosity at low rates of shear by surface active substances: A new hemorheologic phenomenon." *Biorheology* 5 (3), p. 299.

Ehrly, A. M. and B. Lange (1971). "Reduction in blood viscosity and disaggregation of erythrocyte aggregate by streptokinase." In *Theoretical and Clinical Hemorheology*, H. Hartert and A. L. Copley, (Eds.), (1971), p. 366.

Ehrly, A. M. (1971). "Disaggregation of erythrocyte aggregates and decrease of the structural viscosity of human blood by 2-phenyl-benzyl-aminomethyl imidazolidine (antozolin)." In *Theoretical and Clinical Hemorheology*, H. Hartert and A. L. Copley (Eds.), (1971), p. 184.

Einstein, A. (1906). "A new consideration of molecular dimensions" (in German). *Ann. Phys. (Leipzig)* 18, p. 289.

Eiseman, B. and F. C. Spencer (1962). "Effect of hypothermia on the flow characteristics of blood." *Surgery* 52, p. 532.

Eisenberg, S. (1964). "Changes in blood viscosity, hematocrit value and fibrinogen concentration in subjects with congestive heart failure." *Circulation* 30, p. 686.

Eisenberg, S. (1966). "Blood viscosity and fibrinogen concentration following cerebral infarction." *Circulation* 33, p. 10.

Erslev, A. J. and J. Atwater (1963). "Effect of mean corpuscular hemoglobin concentration on viscosity." *J. Lab. Clin. Med.* 62, p. 401.

Engeset, J., A. L. Stalker, and N. A. Matheson (1967a). "Effects of dextran 40 on red cell aggregation in rabbits." *Cardiovasc. Res.* 1 (4), p. 379.

Engeset, J., A. L. Stalker, and N. A. Matheson (1967b). "Objective measurements of the dispersing effect of dextran 40 on red cells from man, dog and rabbit." *Cardiovasc. Res.* 1, p. 385.

Evans, A., J. P. A. Weaver, and D. N. Walder (1967). "A viscometer for the study of blood." *Biorheology* 4, p. 169.

Ewald, C. (1877). "Über die Transpiration des Blutes." *Arch. Anat. Physiol.* 208, p. 32.

Fahey, J. L. (1963). "Serum protein disorders causing clinical symptoms in malignant neoplastic disease." *J. Chron. Dis.* 16, p. 703.

Fahey, J. L., W. F. Barth, and A. Solomon (1965). "Serum hyperviscosity syndrome." *JAMA* 192, p. 464.

Fahraeus, R. (1928). *Klin. Wochenschr.* 7, p. 100. Cited from R. Fahraeus (1929).

Fahraeus, R. (1929). "The suspension stability of the blood." *Physiol. Rev.* 9 (2), p. 241.

Fahraeus, R. and R. Lindquist (1931). "Viscosity of blood in varrow capillary tubes." *Am. J. Physiol.* 96, p. 562.

Fajers, C. M. and L. E. Gelin (1959). "Kidney, liver and heart damages from trauma and from induced intravascular aggregation of blood cells: Experimental study." *Acta Path. Microbiol. Scand.* 46, p. 97.

Finch, C. A. (1972). "Pathophysiologic aspects of sickle-cell anemia." *Am. J. Med.* 53, p. 1.

Fitz-Gerald, J. M. (1969). "Implications of a theory of erythrocyte motion in a narrow capillary." *J. Appl. Physiol.* 27, (6), p. 912.

Fitz-Gerald, J. M. (1972). "The mechanics of capillary blood flow." In *Cardiovascular Fluid Dynamics*, Vol. 2, D. H. Bergel (Ed.). Academic Press, London, p. 205.

Frasher, W. G., H. Wayland, and H. J. Meiselman (1967). "Outflow viscometry in native blood." *Bibl. Anat.* 9, p. 266. Karger, Basel/New York.

Frasher, W. G., H. J. Meiselman, and H. Wayland (1971). "A variable shear rate capillary viscometer for outflow viscometry in dogs." In *Theoretical and Clinical Hemorheology* H. Hartert and A. L. Copley (Eds.), (1971), p. 375.

Freis, E. D., J. R. Stanton, and C. H. P. Emerson (1949). "Estimation of relative velocities of plasma and red cells in circulation of man." *Am. J. Physiol.* 157, p. 153.

Friedman, M., S. O. Byers, and R. H. Rosenman (1965). "Effect of unsaturated fats upon lipemia and conjunctival circulation." *JAMA* 193, p. 110.

Friedman, M., R. H. Rosenman, and S. Byers (1964). "Serum lipids and conjunctival circulation after fat ingestion in men exhibiting type-A behavior pattern." *Circulation* 29, p. 874.

Fukada, E., T. Ibe, K. Atsumi, and T. Osawa (1968). "Viscosity of blood with respect to clinical diagnosis." In *Hemorheology*, A. L. Copley (Ed.), (1968), p. 729.

Fulton, G. P., R. G. Jackson, and B. R. Lutz (1946). "Cinephotomicroscopy of normal blood circulation in the cheek pouch of the hamster, crietus auratus." *Anat. Rec.* 96, p. 537.

Fung, Y. C. (1973). "Stochastic flow in capillary blood vessels." *Microvasc. Res.* 5, p. 34.

Fung, Y. C., B. W. Zweifach, and M. Intagbetta (1966). "Elastic environment of the capillary bed." *Circ. Res.* 19, p. 441.

Fung, Y. C. and S. S. Soliur (1969). "Theory of sheet flow in lung alveoli." *J. Appl. Physiol.* 26, p. 4.

Gaehtgens, P., H. J. Meiselman, and H. Wayland (1969). "Evaluation of the photometric double-slit velocity measuring method in tubes 25 to 30 μ bore." In *5th European Conference on Microcirculation, Gothenburg*. Karger, Basel, p. 571.

Gaehtgens, P., H. J. Meiselman, and H. Wayland (1970). "Erythrocyte flow velocities in mesenteric microvessels of the cat." *Microvasc. Res.* 2, p. 151.

Gaehtgens, P., H. Wayland, and H. J. Meiselman (1971). "Velocity profile measurements in living microvessels by a correlation method." In *Theoretical and Clinical Hemorheology*, H. Hartert and A. L. Copley (Eds.), (1971), p. 381.

Gaisbock, I. (1922). "Die Polyzthamie." *Ergeb. Inn. Med. Kinderheilk* 21, p. 204.

Galluzzi, N. J., R. E. Delashmutt, and V. J. Connolly (1964). "Failure of anticoagulants to influence the viscosity of whole blood." *J. Lab. Clin. Med.* 64, p. 773.

Gelin, L. E. (1961). "Disturbances of the flow properties of blood and its counteraction in surgery." *Acta Clin. Scand.* 122, p. 287.

Gelin, L. E. and B. Lofstrom (1954). "A pulmonary study on peripheral circulation during deep hypothermia." *Acta Clin. Scand.* 108, p. 402.

Gelin, L. E. (1956). "Studies in anemia of injury." *Acta Clin. Scand.* (Suppl.) 210, pp. 1–130.

Gelin, L. E. (1959). "The significance of intravascular aggregation of blood cells following injury." *Bull. Soc. Int. Chirg.* 18, p. 4.

Gelin, L. E. and O. K. A. Thoren (1961). "Influence of low viscous dextran on peripheral circulation in man." *Acta Clin. Scand.* 122, p. 303.

Gelin, L. E. (1963). "A method for studies of aggregation of blood cells, erythrostasis and plasma skimming in branch capillary tubes." *Biorheology* 1, p. 119.

Gelin, L. E., S. E. Bergentz, G. C. Helander, E. Linder, N. J. Nilsson, and C. M. Rudenstam (1968). "Hemodynamic consequences from increased viscosity of blood." In *Hemorheology*, A. L. Copley (Ed.), (1968), p. 721.

Gelin, L. E., J. Kerstell, and A. Svanborg (1967). "The effect of dieting fat on whole blood and plasma viscosity in normal and hypercholesterolemic subjects." *Acta Med. Scand.* 18 (1), p. 41.

Gelin, L. E. (1971). "Rheological effects of dextran." In *"Dextrans – Current Concepts of Basic Actions and Clinical Applications."* J. R. Derrick and M. M. Guest (Eds.), Charles C. Thomas, Springfield, Ill., 1971, Chapter 3.

Gibson, W., P. Bosley, and R. Griffiths (1956). "Photomicrographic studies on the nail bed capillary networks in human control subjects." *J. Nerv. Ment. Dis.* 123, p. 219.

Giombi, A. and E. D. Burnard (1970). "Rheology of human foetal blood with references to hematocrit, plasma viscosity, osmolality and pH." *Biorheology* 6, p. 315.

Glasstone, S. (1946). *Physical Chemistry.* Van Nostrand-Reinhold, New York, p. 260.

Goldsmith, H. J. and S. G. Mason (1961). "Axial migration of particles in Poiseuille flow." *Nature* 190, p. 1095.

Goldsmith, H. J. and S. G. Mason (1962). "The flow of suspension through tubes. 1. Single spheres, rods and discs." *J. Colloid Sci.* 17, p. 448.

Goldsmith, H. L. (1972). "Flow and deformation in human blood: Erythrocytes in ghost cell suspensions." First International Meeting of Biorheology, Lyon, France, September 1972.

Goldsmith, H. L. (1967). "Microscopic flow properties of red cells." *Fed. Proc.* 26 (6), p. 1813.

Goldsmith, H. L. (1968). Personal communication.

Goldsmith, H. L. and S. G. Mason (1971). "Some model experiments in hemodynamics IV." In *Theoretical and Clinical Hemorheology*, H. Hartert and A. L. Copley (Eds.), (1971), p. 47.

Goldstein, S. (1938). In *Modern Developments in Fluid Dynamics*, 2 vols. Clarendon Press, Oxford.

Goldstone, J., H. Schmid-Schönbein, and R. Wells (1970). "Rheoscope – A description of rouleaux breakdown under shear." *Microvasc. Res.* 2, p. 273.

Gordon, W. (1969). "The effect of ingested glucose, and intravenous injections of glucose, on the viscosity of whole blood in man." *Clin. Sci.* 36, p. 25.

Guoy, L. (1910). "Constitution of the electric charge at the surface of an electrolyte." *J. Phys. (Paris)* 2, p. 457.

Gousios, A. and M. A. Shearn (1959). "Effect of intravenous heparin on human blood viscosity." *Circulation* 20, p. 1063.

Gow, B. S. (1972). "Influence of vascular smooth muscle." In *Cardiovascular Fluid Dynamics*, Vol. 2, D. H. Bergel (Ed.). Academic Press, London.

Greenblatt, M., K. V. R. Choudari, A. G. Sanders, and P. Shubik (1960). "Mammalian microcirculation in the living animal: Methodologic considerations." *Microvasc. Res.* 1, p. 420.

Gregersen, M. I. (1971). "Effects of artificial expander agents in blood viscosity." In *"Dextrans – Current Concepts of Basic Actions and Clinical Applications,"* J. R. Derrick and M. M. Guest (Eds.), Charles C. Thomas, Springfield, Ill., 1971, Chapter 2.

Gregersen, M. I., P. Branko, S. Chien, S. Duncan, C. Chang, and H. Taylor (1965). "Viscosity of blood at low shear rates: Observations on its relation to volume concentration and size of red cells." In *Symposium on Biorheology*, A. L. Copley (Ed.), (1965), p. 613.

Gregersen, M. I., C. A. Bryant, W. E. Hammerle, S. Usami, and S. Chien (1967). "Flow characteristics of human erythrocytes through polycarbonate sieves." *Science* 157 (3790), p. 825.

Gregg, D. E. and L. E. Fisher (1963). "Blood supply to the ear." *Circulation* 2, p. 1547.

Gregg, D. E. and H. D. Green (1940). "The effects of viscosity, ischemia, cardiac output and aortic pressure on coronary blood flow measured under constant perfusion pressure." *Am. J. Physiol.* 130, p. 108.

Grillo, G. P. and R. F. Slechta (1963). "Flow rates in small blood vessels of the retrolingual membrane of the frog." *Am. Zool.* 3, 543.

Gross, J. F. and J. Aroesty (1972) "Mathematical models of capillary flow: A critical review." *Biorheology* 9 (4), p. 225.

Groth, G. G. (1965). *Disturbances in the Flow Properties of Blood.* Karolinsks Institute Serafirmerlasarettet, Stockholm, Sweden.

Groth, G. G. (1968). "Plasma expanders and the flow properties of blood." In *Hemorheology*, A. L. Copley (Ed.), (1968), p. 445.

Grotte, G. (1956). "Passage of dextran molecules across the blood–lymph barrier." *Acta Clin. Scand.* **211**, p. 1.

Guest, M., J. R. Derrick, and T. P. Bond (1971). "Altered rheology in human microcirculation resulting from abnormal erythrocytes." *Biorheology* **8**, p. 59.

Guest, M., M. M. Bond, and J. R. Derrick (1963). "Red blood cells: Change in shape of capillaries." *Science* **142**, p. 1319.

Guyton, A. C. and T. O. Richardson (1961). "Effect of hematocrit on venous return." *Circ. Res.* **9**, p. 157.

Hagenbach, E. (1860). "Über die Bestimmung der Zahigkeit einer Flussigkeit durch Ausfluss aus Rohren." *Pogg. Ann.* **109** (385), p. 42.

Hall, C. A. (1965). "Gaisbock's disease: Redefinition of an old syndrome." *Arch. Int. Med.* **116**, p. 4.

Ham, A. W. and T. S. Leeson (1961). *Histology*, 4th ed. Lippincott, Philadelphia.

Ham, T. H. and W. B. Castle (1940). "Relation of increased hypotonic fragility and erythrostasis to the mechanisms of hemolysis in certain anemias." *Trans. Assoc. Am. Physicians* **50**, p. 127.

Ham, T. H., R. T. Dunn, R. W. Sayre, and J. R. Murphy (1968). "Physical properties of red cells as related to effects *in vivo*" *Blood* **32** (6), p. 847.

Hansen, A. T. (1961). "Osmotic pressure effects of the red blood cells – Possible physiological significance." *Nature* **190**, p. 504.

Harkness, J., W. Somerset, and R. B. Whittington (1967). "Variations of human plasma and serum viscosities with their protein content." In *Proc. 4th Europ. Conf. Microcir.*, Cambridge, 1966; *Bibl. Anat.* **9**, p. 226; Karger, Basel–New York.

Harris, J. W. (1950). "Studies in the destruction of red blood cells. VIII. Molecular orientation in sickle-cell hemoglobin solutions." *Proc. Soc. Ex. Biol. Med.* **75**, p. 197.

Harris, J. W., H. H. Brewster, T. H. Ham, and W. B. Castle (1956). "Studies in the destruction of red blood cells – The biophysics and biology of sickle-cell disease." *Arch. Int. Med.* **97**, p. 145.

Harris, P. and D. Heath (1962). *The Human Pulmonary Circulation: Its Form and Function in Health and Disease.* Livingstone, London.

Hartert, H. and A. L. Copley (Eds.) (1971). *Theoretical and Clinical Hemorheology: Proceedings of the Second International Conference on Hemorheology, Heidelberg, Germany.* Springer, New York.

Hatschek, E. (1920). *Koll. Z.* **27**, p. 163. Cited from Bayliss (1952).

Haynes, R. H. and A. C. Burton (1959). "Role of the non-Newtonian behavior of blood in hemodynamics." *Am. J. Physiol.* **197**, p. 943.

Haynes, R. H. and A. C. Burton (1959a). "Axial accumulation of cells and the rheology of blood." *Proc. Nat. Biophys. Conf.*, Columbus, Ohio, p. 452.

Haynes, R. H. and A. C. Burton (1959b). "Role of the non-Newtonian behavior of blood in hemodynamics." *Am. J. Physiol.* **197**, p. 943.

Haynes, R. H. (1960). "Physical basis of the dependence of blood viscosity on tube radius." *Am. J. Physiol.* **198** (3), p. 1193.

Haynes, R. H. (1962). "Arterial and arteriolar systems, biophysical principles." In *Blood Vessels and Lymphatics*, D. J. Abramson (Ed.). Academic Press, New York, p. 26.

Hecht, H. (1971). "A sea level view of altitude problems." *Am. J. Med.* **50**, p. 703.

Heimbecker, R. O. and W. G. Bigelow (1950). "Intravascular agglutination of erythrocytes (sludged blood) and traumatic shock." *Surgery* **28**, p. 461.

Heimberger, H. (1926). "Kontrakile function and anatomischer Basa der menschlichen Kapillaren." *Z. Zellforsch.* **4**, p. 713.

Hellberg, K., H. Wayland, A. L. Rickart, and R. J. Bing (1972). "Studies on the coronary circulation by direct visualization." *Am. J. Cardiol.* **29**, p. 593.

Helmholz, H. (1897). "Studien über elektrische Crenzchichten." *Ann. Phys. Chem.* **7**, p. 337.

Helps, E. P. W. and D. A. McDonald (1954). "Streamline flow in veins." *J. Physiol.* **126**, p. 5.

Herschel, W. H. and R. Bulkley (1926). *Koll. Z.* **39**, p. 291. Cited from *Elementary Rheology*, G. W. Scott-Blair (Ed.). Academic Press, London, 1969.

Hershberg, P. I., R. E. Wells, and R. B. McGandy (1972). "Hematocrit and prognosis in patients with acute myocardial infarction." *JAMA* **219**, p. 855.

Hershey, D. and S. J. Cho (1966). "Laminar flow of suspensions (blood): Thickness and effective slip velocity of the film adjacent to the wall." In *Chemical Engineering in Medicine – Chem. Engine Progress.* Symposium on Biomedical Engineering, American Institute of Chemical Engineers, Philadelphia, p. 139.

Hess, W. R. (1912). Cited from "The emergence of rheology." In H. Marlsovitz, *Phys. Today,* **21** (4), p. 23, 1968.

Hess, W. R. (1920) *Koll. Z.* Cited from Bayliss (1952), p. 1.

Hill, E., G. Power, and L. Longo (1972). "A mathematical model of placental O_2 transfer with consideration of hemoglobin reaction rates." *Am. J. Physiol.* **222** (3), p. 721.

Hint, H. (1971). "Relationships between the chemical and phyicochemical properties of dextran and its pharmacologic effects." In *Dextrans – Current Concepts of Basic Actions and Clinical Applications.* J. R. Derrick, and M. M. Guest (Eds.). Charles C. Thomas, Springfield, Ill., Chapter 1.

Hint, H. and K. E. Arfors (1971). "Specific red cell aggregating activity in normal blood donors and in patients with high sedimentation rate." In *Theoretical and Clinical Hemorheology*, H. Hartert and A. L. Copley (Eds.), (1971), p. 321.

Hint, H. C. (1964). "The flow properties of erythrocyte suspensions in isolated rabbit ear; the effects of erythrocyte aggregation, hematocrit, perfusion pressure." *Bibl. Anat.* **4**, p. 112.

Hochmuth, R. M., R. M. Marple, and S. P. Sutera (1970). "Capillary blood flow. I." *Microvasc. Res.* **2**, p. 409.

Hochmuth, R. and N. Mohandas (1972). "Metabolic dependence of red cell shape: Observation with scanning electron microscope." *Microvasc. Res.,* **4**, p. 295.

Houston, J., R. B. Wittington, I. C. Cowan, and J. Harkness (1949). The plasma viscosity in pulmonary tuberculosis and rheumatic diseases." *J. Clin. Invest.* **28**, p. 752.

Howe, J. T. and Y. S. Scheaffer (1966). "On the dynamics of capillaries and the existence of plasma flow in the pericapillary lymph space." NASA TN-D, 3497.

Huang, K. H. (1971). "Theoretical analysis of flow patterns in single-file capillaries." *J. Biomech.* **4**, p. 103.

224   References

Hübner, W. (1905). "Die Viscosität des Blutes. Bemerkungen zu der gleichnamigen Arbeit von C. Beckund C. Hirsch." *Arch Exp. Path. Pharmalcol.* **54**, p. 149.

Hultgren, H. N. and R. F. Grover (1968). "Circulatory adaptation to high altitude." *Ann. Rev. Med.* **12**, p. 119.

Hyman, W. A. (1973). "The role of slip in the rheology of blood." *Biorheology* **10**, p. 57.

Intaglietta, M. and B. W. Zweifach (1966). "Indirect method for pressure in blood capillaries." *Circ. Res.* **19**, p. 199.

Intaglietta, M. and B. W. Zweifach (1971). "Measurement of blood plasma osmotic pressure, I, II." *Microvasc. Res.* **3**, p. 72.

Irwin, J. W. (1964). "The living microvascular system during anaphylaxis." *Ann. Allerg.* **22**, p. 329.

Isogai, Y., K. Ichiba, I. Chikatsu, and M. Abe (1971). "Viscosity of blood and plasma in various diseases." In *Theoretical and Clinical Hemorheology*, H. Hartert and A. L. Copley (Eds.), (1971), p. 326.

Jacobs, H. R. (1963). "The deformability of red cell packs." *Biorheology* **1** (4), p. 233.

JAMA (1963). "Phlebotomy, an ancient procedure turning modern." A *JAMA* editorial. **183**, p. 279.

Jandl, J. H., R. L. Simmons, and W. B. Castle (1961). "Red cell filtration and the pathogenesis of certain hemolytic anemias." *Blood* **18**, p. 133.

Jasin, H. E., J. LoSpalluto, and M. Ziff (1970). "Rheumatoid hyperviscosity syndrome." *Am. J. Med.* **49**, p. 484.

Jeffery, G. B. (1922). "The motion of ellipsoidal particles immersed in a viscous fluid." *Proc. Roy. Soc., London A* **102**, p. 161.

Johnson, P. C. (1969). "Hemodynamics." *Ann. Rev. Physiol.* **31**, p. 331.

Johnson, P. C. (1972). "Renaissance in the microcirculation." *Circ. Res.* **31** (6), p. 817.

Johnson, P. C. and W. H. Greatbatch, Jr. (1966). "Angiometer: Flying spot microscope for measurement of blood vessel diameter." *Meth. Med. Res.* **11**, p. 220.

Kallio, V., M. Salmivalli, and P. Brummer (1967). "Blood viscosity changes in patients hospitalized because of acute chest pain." *Cardiologia* **50**, p. 323.

Karnovsky, M. J. (1967). "The ultrastructure basis of capillary permeability studied with peroxide as a tracer." *J. Cell. Biol.* **35**, p. 213.

Karnovsky, M. J. (1970). "Morphology of capillaries with special reference to muscle capillaries." In *Capillary Permeability,* C. Crone and N. Lassen, (Eds.). Munksgaard, Copenhagen, p. 331.

Karppinen, K. (1970). "The electrophoretic mobility of red cells and platelets and the plasma viscosity in coronary heart disease." *Acta Med. Scand.* Suppl. 506, p. 7.

Katchalsky, A. and P. F. Curran (1965). *Nonequilibrium Thermodynamics in Biophysics.* Harvard University Press, Cambridge, Mass., p. 119.

Kattus, A. A. and D. E. Gregg (1959). "Some determinants of coronary collateral blood flow in the open-chest dog." *Circ. Res.* **7**, p. 628.

Keen, G. and I. Gerbode (1963). "Observations on the microcirculation during profound hypothemia." *J. Thorac. Cardiovasc. Surg.* **45**, p. 252.

Keitel, H. G., D. Thompson, and H. A. Hano (1956). "Hyposthenuria in sickle-cell anemia: A reversible renal defect." *J. Clin. Invest.* **35**, p. 998.

Kellogg, F. and J. R. Goodman (1960). "Viscosity of blood in myocardial infarction." *Circ. Res.* **8**, p. 972.

Kimmelstein, P. (1948). "Vascular occlusion and ischemic infarction in sickle cell disease." *Am. J. Med.* **216**, p. 11.

Knisely, M. H. (1965). "Intravascular erythrocyte aggregation (blood sludge)." In *Circulation*, Vol. 3, P. Dow (Ed.). American Physiological Society, Washington, D.C., Chapter 63.

Kontras, S., J. Craenen, J. Bodenkender, and D. Hosier (1968). Abstracted in "Hyperviscosity in congenital heart disease." *Circulation* **37/38** (Suppl. 6), p. 118.

Konttinen, A. and T. Somer (1963). "Effect of muscular exercise on plasma viscosity in correlation with postprandial triglyceridemia." *J. Appl. Physiol.* **19**, p. 99.

Kopp, W. L., G. J. Beirne, and R. O. Burns (1967). "Hyperviscosity syndrome in multiple myeloma." *Am. J. Med.* **43**, p. 141.

Kopp, W. L., A. A. MacKinney, Jr., and G. Wasson (1969). "Blood volume and hematocrit in macroglobulinemia and myeloma." *Arch. Int. Med.* **123**, p. 394.

Krieger, I. M. and H. Elrod (1953). *J. Appl. Phys.* **24**, p. 134. Cited from Benis et al. (1971).

Krogh, A. (1922). *The Anatomy and Physiology of Capillaries.* Oxford University Press. London.

Krogh, A. (1919). "The number and distribution of capillaries in muscles with calculations of the oxygen pressure head necessary for supplying." *J. Physiol. (London)* **52** p. 409.

Krovetz, L. J. (1963). "The effects of vessel branching on fluid flow." Ph.D. thesis, University of Minnesota.

Kurland, G. S., S. E. Charm, S. Brown, and P. Tousignant (1968). "Comparison of blood flow in a living vessel and in glass tubes." In *Hemorheology*, A. L. Copley (Ed.), (1968), p. 609.

LaCelle, P. L. (1971). "Erythrocyte deformability and its significance to survival in the microcirculation." In *Theoretical and Clinical Hemorheology,* H. Hartert and A. L. Copley (Eds.), (1971), p. 333.

LaCelle, P. L. and R. I. Weed (1970). "Low oxygen pressure: A cause of erythrocyte membrane rigidity." *J. Clin. Invest.* **49**, p. 54a.

LaCelle, P. L. and R. I. Weed (1972). "The contribution of normal and pathologic erythrocytes to blood rheology." *Progr. Hematol.* **7**, p. 1.

Lamport, H. (1964). "Vascularization compared in thin sheets and blocks of tissue." *Bibl. Anat.* **4**, p. 102.

Landis, E. M. and J. H. Gibbon (1933). "The effects of temperature and of tissue pressure on the movement of fluid through the human wall capillary." *J. Clin. Invest.* **12**, p. 105.

Landis, E. M. and J. R. Pappenheimer (1963). In *Handbook of Physiology – Circulation,* Vol. 2. American Physiological Society, Washington, D.C., p. 961.

Langsjoen, H. (1967). "Rheologic changes in myocardial infarction." *Am. Heart J.* **73**, p. 430.

Laszt, L. and A. Müller (1952). "Uber den Druckverlauf im bereiche der Aorta." *Helv. Physiol. Acta* **10**, p. 1.

Lawrence, J. H. and N. I. Berlin (1952). "Relative polycythemia – Polycythemia of stress." *Yale J. Biol. Med.* **24**, p. 498.

Lee, J. S. and Y. C. Fung, (1969). Modeling experiments of a single red cell moving in a capillary blood vessel." *Microvasc. Res.* 1, p. 221.

Lee, W. H., A. Najib, M. Weidner, G. H. A. Clowes, E. S. Murner, and V. Vujovic (1968). "The significance of apparent blood viscosity in circulatory hemodynamic behavior." In *Hemorheology*, A. L. Copley (Ed.), (1968), p. 587.

Lee, J. L. and Y. C. Fung (1971). "Flow in non-uniform small blood vessels." *Microvasc. Res.* 3, p. 272.

Lessner, A., J. Zahavi, A. Silberberg, E. H. Frei, and F. Dreyfuss (1971). "The viscoelastic properties of whole blood." In *Theoretical and Clinical Hemorheology*, H. Hartert and A. L. Copley (Eds.), (1971), p. 194.

Levitt, M. F., A. D. Hauser, M. S. Levy, and D. Polimeros (1960). "The renal concentrating mechanism in sickle-cell disease." *Am. J. Med.* 29, p. 611.

Levy, M. N. and L. Share (1953). "The influence of erythrocyte concentration upon the pressure flow relationships in the dogs hind limb." *Circ. Res.* 1, p. 247.

Lew, H. S. and Y. C. Fung (1969). "The motion of the plasma between the red cells in the bolus flow." *Biorheology* 6 (2), p. 109.

Lew, H. S. and Y. C. Fung (1969). "On the low-Reynolds-number entry flow into a circular cylindrical tube." *J. Biomech.* 2, p. 105.

Lewis, W. K. and W. G. Whitman (1924). *Ind. Eng. Chem.* 16, p. 1215. Cited from Walker et al., *Principles of Chemical Engineering*, McGraw-Hill, New York, 1937.

Lewy, B. (1897). "Die Reibung des Blutes." *Pflugers Arch.* 65, p. 26.

Lighthill, N. J. (1968). "Pressure-forcing of tightly fitting elastic pellets along fluid-filled elastic tubes." *J. Fluid Mech.* 34, p. 113.

Lindsley, H., B. Noonan, M. Peterson, and M. Mannik (1973). "Hyperviscosity syndrome in myeloma." *Am. J. Med.* 54, p. 682.

Lino, L. and R. L. Swank (1968). "Blood plasma lipids after different meals." In *Hemorheology* A. L. Copley (Ed.), (1968), p. 787.

Litwin, M. S., S. E. Bergentz, A. Carsten, L. A. Gelin, C. M. Rudenstam, and B. Soderholm (1965). "Hidden acidosis following intravascular red blood cell aggregation in dogs. Effects of high-low viscosity dextran." *Ann. Surg.* 161, p. 532.

Long, D. M., Jr., L. Sanchez, R. L. Varco, and C. W. Hillehei (1961). "Use of low molecular weight dextran and serum albumin as plasma expanders in extracorporeal circulation." *Surgery* 50, p. 12.

Luft, J. H. (1966). "Fine structure of capillary and endocapillary layer as revealed by ruthenium red." *Fed. Proc.* 25 (6), p. 1773.

Lundskog, J., P. I. Branemark, J. Lindstrom (1968). "Biomicroscopic evaluation of microangiographic methods." In *Advances of Microcirculation*, H. Harders (Ed.). S. Karger, Basel.

Mack, I. and G. Snider (1966). "Respiratory insufficiency and chronic cor pulmonale." *Circulation* 13, p. 419.

Madow, B. and E. H. Bloch (1956). "Effect of erythrocyte aggregation on rheology of blood." *Angiology* 7, p. 1.

Maggio, E. (1965). *Microhemocirculation*, Charles C. Thomas, Springfield, Ill., p. 78.

Majno, G., V. Gilmore, and M. Leventhal (1967). "On the mechanism of vascular leakage caused by histamine-type mediators." *Circ. Res.* 21, p. 823.

Marticorena, E., L. Ruiz, J. Severino, J. Galvez, and D. Penaloza (1969). "Systemic blood pressure in white men born at sea level: Changes after long residence at high altitudes." *Am. J. Cardiol.* **23**, p. 364.

Marty, A. T., A. J. Eraklios, G. A. Pelletier, and E. W. Merrill (1971). "The rheologic effects of hypothermia on blood with high hematocrit values." *J. Thorac. Cardiovasc. Surg.* **61**, p. 735.

Maude, A. D. and R. L. Whitmore (1956). "The wall effect and the viscometry of suspensions." *Brit. J. Appl. Physiol.* **7**, p. 98.

Maude, A. D. and R. L. Whitmore (1958). "Theory of the flow of blood in narrow tubes." *J. Appl. Physiol.* **12**, p. 105.

May, A., J. DeWeese, and C. Rab (1963). "Hemodynamic effects of arterial stenosis." *Surgery* **53** (1), p. 513.

Mayer, G. A. and O. Kiss (1965). "Blood viscosity and *in vitro* anticoagulants." *Am. J. Physiol.* **208** (4), p. 795.

Mayer, G. A. (1966). "Relation of the viscosity of plasma and whole blood." *Am. J. Clin. Path.* **45**, p. 273.

Mayer, G. A. (1964). "Blood viscosity in healthy subjects and patients with coronary heart disease." *Can. Med. Assoc. J.* **91**, p. 951.

Mayer, G. A., J. Frederick, J. Newell, and J. Szivek (1966). "Plasma components and blood viscosity." *Biorheology* **3**, p. 177.

McCurdy, P. R. and L. Mahmood (1971). "Intravenous urea treatment of the painful crisis of sickle-cell disease." *N. Eng. J. Med.* **285**, p. 992.

McDonald, D. A. (1960). *Blood Flow in Arteries.* Williams & Wilkins, Baltimore, p. 174.

McDonald, D. A. and J. M. Potter (1963). "Blood streams in the basilar artery." Film: 16 mm; color, silent; Wellcome Film Unit. Available on loan from Burroughs, Wellcome Co., Inc., Tuckahoe, N.Y. Noted in Krovetz (1963).

McDonough, J. R., C. G. Hames, G. E. Garrison, S. G. Stulb, M. A. Lichtman, and D. C. Hefelfinger (1965). "The relationship of hematocrit to cardiovascular states of health in the negro and white population of Evans County, Georgia." *J. Chronic Dis.* **18**, p. 243.

McNamara, J. J., M. D. Molot, and J. F. Stremple (1972). "Blood viscosity in combat casualties." *Surg. Gynecol. Obstetr.* **134**, p. 293.

Meiselman, H., W. Frasher, and H. Wayland (1971). "Variable shear rate viscometry of native blood: Effect of heparin injection." *Biorheology* **8**, p. 98.

Meiselman, H. J., W. G. Frasher, and H. Wayland (1972). "The effects of fibrination on the *in vivo* rheology of dogs' blood." *Microvasc. Res.* **4**, p. 26.

Meiselman, H. J. and E. W. Merrill (1968). "Observations on the rheology of human blood: Effect of low molecular weight dextran." In *Hemorheology*, A. L. Copley (Ed.). (1968), p. 421.

Meiselman, H. J., E. W. Merrill, E. R. Gilliland, G. A. Pelletier, and E. W. Salzman (1967). "Influence of plasma osmolarity on the rheology of human blood." *J. Appl. Physiol.* **22**, p. 772.

Mellander, S. and D. H. Lewis (1963). "Effect of hemorrhagic shock on the reactivity of resistance and capacitance vessels and on capillary filtration in cat skeletal muscle." *Circ. Res.* **13**, p. 105.

Meltzer, M. and E.C. Franklin (1966). "Cryoglobulinemia – A study of 29 patients." *Am. J. Med.* **40**, p. 828.

Mendlowitz, M. (1948). "The effect of anemia and polycythemia on digital intravascular blood viscosity." *J. Clin. Invest.* **27**, p. 565.

Merrill, E. W., E. R. Gilliland, G. Cokelet, H. Shin, A. Britten, and R. E. Wells, Jr. (1963). "Rheology of blood and flow in the microcirculation." *J. Appl. Physiol.* **18**, p. 255.

Merrill, E. W., E. R. Gilliland, T. S. Lee, and E. W. Salzman (1966). "Blood rheology: Effect of fibrinogen deduced by addition." *Circ. Res.* **18**, p. 437.

Merrill, E. W., E. R. Gilliland, W. G. Margetts, and F. T. Hatch (1964). "Rheology of human blood and hyperlipemia." *J. Appl. Physiol.* **19**, p. 493.

Merrill, E. W. and R. E. Wells (1961). "Flow properties of biological fluids." *Appl. Mech. Rev.* **14**, p. 663.

Merrill, E. W., E. R. Gilliland, G. R. Cokelet, H. Shin, A. Britten, and R. E. Wells (1963a). "Rheology of human blood: Effect of temperature and hematocrit." *Biophys. J.* **3**, p. 199.

Merrill, E. W., G. R. Cokelet, A. Britten, and R. E. Wells (1963b). "Non-Newtonian rheology of human blood: Effect of fibrinogen deduced by subtraction." *Circ. Res.* **13**, p. 48.

Merrill, E. W., G. Cokelet, A. Britten, and R. E. Wells (1964). "Rheology of human blood and the red cell plasma membrane." *Bibl. Anat.* **4**. Karger, New York, p. 51.

Merrill, E. W., A. M. Benis, A. R. Gilliland, T. K. Sherwood, and E. W. Salzman (1965a). "Pressure–flow relations of human blood in hollow fibers at low flow rates." *J. Appl. Physiol.* **20** (5), p. 954.

Merrill, E. W., W. G. Margetts, G. R. Cokelet, and E. R. Gilliland (1965b). The Casson equation and rheology of blood near zero shear." In *Symposium on Biorheology*, A. L. Copley (Ed.), (1965), p. 135.

Merrill, E. W. and G. A. Pelletier (1967). "Viscosity of human blood: Transition from Newtonian to non-Newtonian." *J. Appl. Physiol.* **33**, p. 178.

Merrill, E. W. (1969). "Rheology of blood." *Physiol. Rev.* **49**, p. 863.

Michel, C. C. (1972). "Flow across the capillary wall." In *Cardiovascular Fluid Dynamics*, Vol. 2. D. H. Bergel (Ed.). Academic Press, London, p. 242.

Middleman, S. (1972). *Transport Phenomena in the Cardiovascular System.* Interscience, New York, p. 127.

Miller, A. T., Jr. and D. M. Hale (1970). "Increased vascularity of brains, heart and skeletal muscle of polycythemic rats." *Am. J. Physiol.* **219**, p. 702.

Millikan, C. H., R. G. Siekert, and J. P. Whisnant (1960). "Intermittent carotid and vertebral gasilar insufficiency associated with polycythemia." *Neurology* **10**, p. 188.

Mitvalsky, V. (1965). "Heat transfer in laminar flow of human blood through tube and annuli." *Nature* (4981), p. 307.

Mohandas, N., R. M. Hochmuth, and J. R. Williamson (1972). "Deformation of red cells adhering to surfaces." Seventh Conference on Microcirculation (Abstract), Aberdeen, Scotland.

Monro, P. A. G. (1963). "The appearance of cell-free plasma and "grouping" of red blood cells in normal circulation in small blood vessels observed *in vivo*." *Biorheology* **1**, p. 239.

Monro, P. A. G. (1965). "Visual particle velocity measurements in fluid streams." In *Symposium on Biorheology*, A. Copley (Ed.), (1965), p. 439.

Mooney, M. (1931). "Explicit formulas for slip and fluidity." *J. Rheol.* 2, p. 210.

Moskow, H. A., R. C. Pennington, and M. H. Knisely (1968). "Alcohol sludge and hypoxic areas of nervous system, liver and heart." *Microvasc. Res.* 1, p. 174.

Mostofi, F. K., C. F. Bruegge, and L. W. Diggs (1967). "Lesions in kidney removed for unilateral hematuria in sickle-cell disease." *Arch. Path.* 63, p. 336.

Muller, A. (1941). *Arch. Kreisl. Forsch.* 8, p. 245. Cited from *Deformation and Flow in Biological Systems*, A. Frey-Wyssling (Ed.). Interscience, New York, 1952, p. 367.

Murphy, J. R. (1968). "Erythrocyte shape and blood viscosity." In *Hemorheology*, A. L. Copley (Ed.), (1968), p. 469.

Murphy, J. R. (1968). "Hemoglobin CC disease: Rheologic properties of erythrocytes and abnormalities in cell water." *J. Clin. Invest.* 47, p. 1483.

Murray, J. F., E. Esobar, and E. Rapaport (1969). "Effects of blood viscosity on hemodynamic responses in acute normovolemic anemia." *Am. J. Physiol.* 216, p. 638.

Nashat, F. S., F. R. Scholefield, S. W. Rappin, and C. S. Wilcox (1969). "The effects of changes in hematocrit on the intrarenal distribution of blood flow in the dog's kidney." *J. Physiol.* 201, p. 639.

Navar, R. M. and J. L. Gainer (1968). "Prediction of the sigma effect in blood flow." *Biorheology* 5 (3), p. 237.

Nee, W. H., Jr., A. Najib, M. Weidner, G. Clowes, E. S. Murner, and V. Vujovic (1969). "The significance of apparent blood viscosity in circulatory hemodynamic behavior." In *Hemorheology*, A. L. Copley (Ed.), (1968), p. 587.

Nims, J. C. and J. W. Irwin (1973). "Chamber techniques to study the microvasculature." *Microvasc. Res.* 5, p. 105.

Nubar, Y. (1966). "The laminar flow of a composite fluid: An approach to the rheology of blood." *Ann. N.Y. Acad. Sci.* 136 (art. 2), p. 33.

Nubar, Y. (1967). "Effect of slip on the rheology of a composite fluid: Application to blood." *Biorheology* 4, p. 113.

Oka, S. (1971). "An approach to a unified theory of flow behavior of time independent non-Newtonian suspensions." *Jap. J. Appl. Physics* 10 (3), p. 287.

Oscai, L. B., B. T. Williams, and B. A. Hertig (1968). "Effect of exercise on blood volume." *J. Appl. Physiol.* 24 (5), p. 662.

Ossoff, R. and Charm S. E. (1972). "Blood flow in charged polyelectrolyte capillary tubes." First International Conference on Biorheology, Lyon, France., September 1972.

Palade, G. E. (1968). "Small pore and large pore systems in capillary permeability." In *Hemorheology*, A. L. Copley (Ed.), (1968), p. 703.

Palmer, A. A. (1959). "A study of blood flow in minute vessels of the pancreatic region of the rate with reference to intermittent corpuscular flow in individual capillaries." *Quart. J. Exp. Physiol.* 44, p. 149.

Palmer, A. A. (1965). "Axial drift of cells and partial plasma skimming in blood flowing through glass slits." *Am. J. Physiol.* 206 (6), p. 1115.

Palmer, A. A. (1971). "The influence of the length of a capillary channel on the axial accumulation of red cells." In *Theoretical and Clinical Hemorheology*, H. Hartert and A. L. Copley (Eds.), (1971), p. 213.

Palmer, A. A, and W. Betts (1972). "The influence of flow rate and hematocrit on the location of the zone of maximum cell concentration in blood flowing down a capillary." First International Congress of Biorheology, Lyon, France, September 1972.

Palmer, A. A. and W. H. Betts (1972). "The influence of plasma skimming and axial drift of red cells." Seventh Conference on Microcirculation, Aberdeen, Scotland, 1972. (Abstract).

Pappenheimer, J. R., E. M. Renkin, L. M. Borrero (1951). "Filtration, diffusion and molecular sieving through peripheral capillary membranes." *Am. J. Physiol.* **167**, p. 13.

Penaloza, D. and Francisco, S. (1971). "Chronic cor pulmonale due to loss of altitude acclimatization." *Am. J. Med.* **50**, p. 728.

Perl, W. (1971). "Modified filtration–permeability model of transcapillary transport – A solution of the Pappenheimer pore puzzle." *Microvasc. Res.* **3**, p. 233.

Perry, J. H. (1963). In *Chemical Engineers Handbook*, 4th ed. McGraw-Hill, New York, p. 5.

Phibbs, R. H. (1966). "Distribution of leukocytes in blood flowing through arteries." *Am. J. Physiol.* **210**, p. 919.

Phibbs, R. H., (1967). "Orientation and distribution of erythrocytes in blood flowing through medium-sized arteries." *Biorheology* **4**, p. 97.

Phibbs, R. H. (1967). Personal communication.

Pirofsky, B. (1953). "The determination of blood viscosity in man by a method based on Poiseuille's law." *J. Clin. Invest.* **32**, p. 292.

Poiseuille, J. L. M. (1835), *C. R. Acad. Sci. Paris* **1**, p. 554. Cited from *Flow Properties of Blood*, A. L. Copley and G. Stainsby (Eds.), Pergamon Press, New York, 1960, p. 422.

Poiseuille, J. L. M. (1842). "Recherches experimentales sur le mouvement des liquides dans les tubes de très-petits diametres." *Compt. Rend.* **15**, p. 1167.

Ponder, E. (1940). "Red cell as osmometer." *Cold Spring Harbor Symp. Quantit. Biol.* **8**, p. 133.

Pories, W. J., P. D. Harris, J. R. Hinshaw, T. P. Davis, and S. I. Schwartz (1962). "Blood sludging: An experimental critique of its occurrence, supposed effects." *Ann. Surg.* **155**, p. 33.

Pringle, R., D. N. Walder, and J. P. A. Weaver (1965). "Blood viscosity and Raynaud's disease." *Lancet* **1**, p. 1086.

Prothero, J. and A. C. Burton (1962). "The physics of blood flow in capillaries. 11. The capillary resistance to flow." *Biophys. J.* **2**, p. 199.

Pruzanski, W. and J. G. Watt (1972). "Serum viscosity and hyperviscosity syndrome in IgG multiple myeloma." *Ann. Int. Med.* **77**, p. 853.

Rabinowitsch, B. (1929). "Über die Viskosetät and Elastizität von Solen." *Z. Phys. Chem.* **2** (A145), p. 1.

Rand, P. W., E. Lacombe, H. E. Hunt, and W. H. Austin (1964). "Viscosity of normal human blood under nonuothormic and hypothermic conditions." *J. Appl. Physiol.* **19**, p. 117.

Rand, P. W., N. Barker, and E. Lacombe (1970). "Effects of plasma viscosity and aggregation in whole blood viscosity." *Am. J. Physiol.* **218**, p. 681.

Rand, R. P. and A. C. Burton (1964). "Mechanical properties of the red cell membrane." *Biophysics J.* **4**, p. 115.

Rand, R. P. (1967). "Some biophysical considerations of the red cell membrane." *Fed. Proc.* **26**, p. 1780.

Rathe, G. (1958). "Relacion entre viscosidad relativa de la sangre y concentracion, tamario y forma de los eritrocitos." *Rev. Soc. Arg. Biol.* **34**, p. 1.

Rees, S. B., L. Simon, and G. A. Peltier (1968). "Hemorheologic studies during the progression and remission of diabetic retinopathy." Abstracted in *Hemorheology*, A. L. Copley (Ed.), (1968), p. 763.

Regan, T. J., K. Binak, S. Gordon, V. DeFazio, and H. K. Hellems (1959). "The modification of myocardial blood flow and oxygen consumption during postprandial lipemia and leparin induced lipolysis." *J. Clin. Invest.* **38**, p. 1033.

Regan, T. J., M. J. Frank, P. H. Lehan, and H. K. Hellems (1960). "Influence of red cell mass on myocardial blood flow and oxygen uptake." *Clin. Res.* **8**, p. 367.

Regan, T. J., G. Timmis, M. Gray, K. Binak, and H. K. Hellems (1961). "Myocardial oxygen consumption during exercise in fasting and lipemic subjects." *J. Clin. Invest.* **40**, p. 624.

Regan, T. J., M. J. Frank, P. H. Lehan, J. G. Galante, and H. K. Hellems (1963). "Myocardial blood flow and oxygen uptake during acute red cell volume increments." *Circ. Res.* **13**, p. 172.

Reiner, M. and G. Scott-Blair (1958). "The importance of the sigma phenomenon in the study of the flow of blood." *Rheolog. Acta* **1** (2–3).

Reiner, M. and G. Scott-Blair (1959). "The flow of blood through narrow tubes." *Nature*, **184**, p. 354.

Repetti, R. and E. F. Leonard (1966). "Physical basis for the axial accumulation of red blood cells." *Chem. Eng. Progr. Symp. Ser.* **62**, p. 80.

Replogle, R. L., H. Kundler, and R. E. Gross (1965). "Studies on the hemodynamic importance of blood viscosity." *J. Thorac. Cardiovasc. Surg.* **50**, p. 658.

Replogle, R. L., H. H. Meiselman, and E. W. Merrill (1967). "Clinical implications of blood rheology studies." *Circulation* **36**, p. 148.

Reubi, F. C. (1953). "Glomerular filtration rate, renal blood flow and blood viscosity during and after diabetic coma." *Circ. Res.* **1**, p. 410.

Richardson, T. G. and A. C. Gayton (1959). "Effects of polycythemia and anemia on cardiac output and other circulatory factors." *Am. J. Physiol.* **197**, p. 1167.

Riley, R. L. (1965). "Gas exchange and transportation." In *Physiology and Biophysics*, Ruch and Patton (Eds.). Saunders Philadelphia, p. 765.

Rosenblatt, G., J. Stokes and D. R. Bassett (1965). "Whole blood viscosity, hematocrit and serum lipid levels in normal subjects and patients with coronary heart disease." *J. Lab. Clin. Med.* **65**, p. 202.

Rosenblum, W. I. (1968). "*In vitro* measurements of the effects of anticoagulants on the flow properties of blood: The relationship of these effects to red cell shrinkage." *Blood* **31** (2), p. 234.

Rosenblum, W. I. and R. M. Asofsky (1968a). "Malfunction of cerebral circulation in macroglobulinemic mice." *Arch. Neurol.* **18**, p. 151.

Rosenblum, W. I. and R. M. Asofsky (1968b). "Factors affecting blood viscosity in macroglobulinemic mice." *J. Lab. Clin. Med.* **71**, p. 201.

Rosenblum, W. I. (1969). "Vasoconstriction, blood viscosity and erythrocyte aggregation in macroglobulinemic and polycythemic mice." *J. Lab. Clin. Med.* **73**, p. 359.

Rosenblum, W. I. (1970). "The differential effect of elevated blood viscosity on plasma and erythrocyte flow in the cerebral microcirculation of the mouse." *Microvasc. Res.* 2, p. 399.

Rosenblum, W. I. (1970). "Effects of blood pressure and blood viscosity on fluorescein transit time in the cerebral microcirculation in the mouse." *Circ. Res.* 27, p. 825.

Rosenblum, W. I. and E. W. Warren (1973). "Elevation of blood viscosity produced by shearing in a rotational viscometer and its inhibition by refrigeration." *Biorheology* 10, p. 43.

Rosenthal, A., D. C. Nathan, A. T. Marty, L. N. Button, O. S. Miettn, and A. Nadas (1970). "Acute hemodynamic effects of red cell volume reduction in polycythemia of congenital heart disease." *Circulation* 42, p. 297.

Roughton, F. J. W. (1963). "Kinetics of gas transport in blood." *Brit. Med. Bull.* 19, p. 80.

Roughton, F. J. W. and R. E. Forster (1957). "Relative importance of diffusion and chemical reaction rates in determining rates of exchange of gases in the human lung with special reference to the true diffusing capacity of pulmonary membrane and volume of blood in the lung capillaries." *J. Appl. Physiol.* 11, p. 290.

Rowe, G., D. McKenna, R. Corliss, and S. Sialer (1972). "Hemodynamic effects of hypertonic sodium chloride." *J. Appl. Physiol.* 32, p. 182.

Rowlands, S., A. C. Groom, and H. W. Thomas (1965). "The difference in circulation times between erythrocytes and plasma *in vivo*." In *Symposium on Biorheology*, A. L. Copley (Ed.), (1965), p. 371.

Rubinow, S. I. and J. B. Keller (1961). "The transverse force on a spinning sphere moving in a viscous liquid." *J. Fluid Mech.* 11, p. 447.

Ruch, T. C. and Patton (1965). *Physiology and Biophysics*, W. B. Saunders, Philadelphia, p. 1053.

Rudolph, A. M., A. S. Nadas, and W. H. Borges (1953). "Hematologic adjustments to cyanotic congenital heart disease." *Pediatrics* 11, p. 454.

Rumscheidt, F. D. and S. G. Mason (1961). "Particle motions in sheared suspensions. XII. Deformation and burst of fluid drops in shear and hyperbolic flow." *J. Colloid Sci.* 16, p. 238.

Russel, R. P. and C. L. Conley (1964). "Benign polycythemia: Gaisbock's syndrome." *Arch. Int. Med.* 114, p. 734.

Saffman, P. G. (1956). "On the motion of small spheroidal particles in a viscous fluid." *J. Fluid Mech.* 1, p. 540.

Saperstein, L. (1958). *The Microcirculation*, University of Illinois Press, Urbana, p. 48.

Sawyer, P. N. and E. H. Himmelfarb (1965). "Studies of streaming potential in large mammalian blood vessels *in vivo*." In *Biophysical Mechanisms in Vascular Homeostasis and Intravascular Thrombosis*, Sawyer (Ed.). Appleton-Century Crofts, New York, p. 75.

Scatchard, G., A. C. Batchelder, and A. Brown (1946). "Preparation and properties of serum and plasma proteins. IV. Osmotic equilibria in solutions of serum albumin and sodium chloride." *J. Am. Chem. Soc.* 68, p. 2320.

Schenk, E. A. (1964). "Sickle-cell trait and superior longitudinal sinus thrombosis." *Ann. Int. Med.* 60, p. 465.

Schlichting, H. (1960). In *Boundary Layer Theory*, J. Kestin (Ed.), McGraw-Hill, New York, p. 21.

Schlitt, L. E. and L. G. Keitel (1960). "Renal manifestation of sickle-cell disease: A review." *Am. J. Med. Sci.* **239**, p. 773.

Schmid-Schönbein, H., P. Gaehtgens, and H. Hirsch (1968). "On the shear rate dependence of red cell aggregation *in vitro*." *J. Clin. Invest.* **47**, p. 1447.

Schmid-Schönbein, H., R. Wells, and J. Goldstone (1969). "Influence of deformability of human red cells upon blood viscosity." *Circ. Res.* **25**, p. 131.

Schmid-Schönbein, H., J. Goldstone, and R. Wells (1971a). "Model experiment in red cell rheology; The mammalian erythrocyte as a fluid drop." In *Theoretical and Clinical Hemorheology,*" H. Hartert and A. L. Copley (Eds.), (1971), p. 233.

Schmid-Schönbein, H. and R. Wells (1971b). "Red cell aggregation and red cell deformation: Their influence on blood rheology in health and disease." In *Theoretical and Clinical Hemorheology*, H. Hartert and A. L. Copley (Eds.), (1971), p. 348.

Schmid-Schönbein, H., J. Van Gosen, and H. Klose (1972). "Comparative microbiology of blood: Effect of disaggregation red cell orientation and red cell fluidity on shear thinning of blood in various species." First International Conference of Biorheology, Lyon, France, September 1972.

Schmidt-Nielsen, K., and C. R. Taylor (1968). "Red blood cells: Why or why not?" *Science* **162**, p. 274.

Schwartz, T. B. and R. I. Apfelbaum (1965–1966) "Nonketotic diabetic coma." In *Year Book of Endocrinology*, Year Book Medical Publishers, Chicago, p. 165.

Scott-Blair, G. W. (1960). "Note on the sigma phenomenon." *Am. J. Physiol.* **199**, p. 1245.

Scott-Blair, G. W. (1968). "Basic equations for flow of blood through an artificial capillary and for fibrin polymerization and softening." In *Hemorheology*, A. L. Copley (Ed.), (1968), p. 345.

Scott-Blair, G. W. (1967a). *Rheolog. Acta.* Cited in July 1968 issue of *Biorheology*, **5** (2), p. 22.

Scott-Blair, G. W. (1967b). "A model to describe the flow curves of concentrated suspensions of spherical particles." *Rheolog. Acta* **6**, p. 201.

Seaman, G. V. F. and R. L. Swank (1967). "The influence of electrokinetic charge and deformability of the red blood cell on the flow properties of its suspensions." *Biorheology* **4**, p. 47.

Sedziwy, L., J. Shillingford, and M. Thomas (1968). "Some observations on hematocrit changes in patients with acute myocardial infarction." *Brit. Heart J.* **30**, p. 344.

Segel, N. and J. M. Bishop (1966). "Circulation in patients with chronic bronchitis and emphysema at rest and during exercise, with special reference to the influence of changes in blood viscosity and blood volume on the pulmonary circulation." *J. Clin. Invest.* **45**, p. 1555.

Segre, G. and A. Silberberg (1962a). "Behavior of macroscopic rigid spheres in Poiseuille flow. Parts 1 and 2." *J. Fluid Mech.* **14**, p. 115.

Segre, G. and A. Silberberg (1962b). "Behavior of macroscopic rigid spheres in Poiseuille flow." *J. Fluid Mech.* **14**, p. 136.

Seligman, A. M., H. A. Frank, and J. Fine (1946). "Traumatic shock. XII. Hemodynamic effects of alterations of blood viscosity in normal dogs and in dogs in shock." *J. Clin. Lab.* **25**, p. 1.

Shapiro, A. H. (1961). *Shape and Flow, the Fluid Dynamics of Drag.* Doubleday, Garden City, N.Y.

Shearn, M. and A. Gousios (1960). "Effect of intravenous fat emulsions on human blood viscosity." *Arch. Int. Med.* **106**, p. 619.

Shearn, M., W. V. Epstein, E. Engleman, and W. F. Taylor (1963). "Relationship of serum proteins and rheumatoid factor to serum viscosity in rheumatic diseases." *J. Lab. Clin. Med.* **61**, p. 677.

Shepro, D. and G. P. Fulton (1968). *Microcirculation as Related to Shock.* Academic Press, New York.

Sheshadri, V. and S. P. Sutera (1968). "Concentration changes of suspensions of rigid spheres flowing through tubes." *J. Colloid Interface Sci.* **27** (1), p. 101.

Shinagawa, T. (1964). "Studies on atherosclerosis, mainly about its relationship with serum viscosity (I)." *Jap. Circ. J.* **28**, p. 324.

Shorrock, J. E. T. and H. Hillman (1969). "The viscosity of rat blood between the temperatures of 2 and 35°C." *Cryobiology* **5**, p. 324.

Shorthouse, B. O. and M. T. Hutchinson (1967). "Investigation into the visco-elasticity of cell free plasma using the Bio-Rheogoniometer." In *4th European Conf. Microcirculation*, Cambridge, 1966. *Bibl. Anat.* **9**, p. 232. Karger, Basel, New York.

Sieder, E. N. and G. E. Tate (1936). *Eng. Chem.* **28**, p. 1429. Cited from *Perry's Handbook of Chemical Engineering*, 4th ed., McGraw-Hill, New York, 1963.

Silberberg, A. (1966). "The tubular pinch effect in the circulation of blood." *Biorheology* **4**, p. 29.

Sirs, J. A. (1968). "The measurement of the hematocrit and flexibility of erythrocytes with a centrifuge." *Biorheology* **5** (1), p. 1.

Skalak, R. and P. I. Branemark (1969). "Deformation of red blood cells in capillaries." *Science* **164**, p. 717.

Skovberg, F., A. V. Nielsen, J. Schlichtkrull, and J. Ditzel (1966). "Blood viscosity in diabetic patients." *Lancet* **1**, p. 129.

Skovborg, F., A. Nielsen, and J. Schlichtkrull (1968). "Blood viscosity and vascular flow rate. Blood viscosity measured in a cone–plate viscometer and the flow rate in an isolated vascular bed." *Scand. J. Clin. Lab. Invest.* **21**, p. 83.

Slechta, R. and G. P. Fulton (1963). "Blood flow rates in small vessels of the hamster cheek pouch." *Proc. Soc. Exp. Biol. Med.* **112**, p. 1076.

Smith, E., J. Kochwas, and L. E. Wasserman (1965). "Aggregation of IgG globulinin *in vivo*. I: The hyperviscosity syndrome in multiple myeloma." *Am. J. Med.* **39**, p. 35.

Sobin, S. S. and H. M. Tremer (1966). "Functional geometry of the microcirculation." *Fed. Proc.* **256**, p. 1744.

Sobin, S. S. and H. M. Tremer (1972). "Diameter of myocardial capillaries." *Microvasc. Res.* **4**, p. 330. (Abstract).

Somer, T. (1966). "The viscosity of blood, plasma and serum in Dys and paraproteinemias." *Acta Med. Scand.* **180**, Suppl. 456.

Stables, D. P., A. H. Rubenstein, J. Metz, and N. W. Levin (1967). "The possible role of hemocirculation in the etiology of myocardial infarction." *Am. Heart J.* **73**, p. 155.

Stalker, A. L. (1964). "Intravascular erythrocyte aggregation." *Bibl. Anat.* **4**, p. 108.

Stehbens, W. E. (1959). "Turbulence and blood flow." *Quart. J. Exp. Physiol.* **44**, p. 110.

Stein, R. R., J. C. Martin, H. K. Keller (1971). "Steady-state oxygen transport through blood cell suspensions." *J. Appl. Physiol.* **31** (3), p. 397.

Steinberg, M. H. and S. E. Charm (1971). "Effect of high concentrations of leukocytes on whole blood viscosity." *Blood* **38**, p. 299.

Stoltz, J. F., M. Stoltz, and A. Larcan (1972). "Action of two polybases on the charge of blood components." Seventh Conference on Microcirculation, Aberdeen, Scotland, 1972.

Stolz, J. F. and A. Larcan (1971). "A method for measuring the electrophoretic mobility of colloidal particles in suspension. Theory and comparison between four different cells." In *Theoretical and Clinical Hemorheology*, H. Hartert and A. L. Copley (Eds.), (1971), p. 388.

Stone, H. O., H. K. Thompson, Jr., and K. Schmidt-Nielsen (1968). "Influence of erythrocytes in blood viscosity." *Am. J. Physiol.* 214, p. 913.

Strike, B. and H. Schmid-Schönbein (1970). Personal communication.

Strumia, M. M. and M. Phillips (1963). "Effect of red cell factors on the relative viscosity of whole blood." *Am. J. Clin. Pathol.* 39, p. 464.

Sutera, S. P. and R. M. Hochmuth (1968). "Large scale modeling of blood in the capillaries." *Biorheology* 5 (1) p. 45.

Sutera, S. P., V. Seshachi, P. A. Coce, and R. N. Hochmuth (1970). "Capillary blood flow. II. Deformable model cells in the tube flow." *Microvasc. Res.* 2, p. 420.

Swank, R. L. (1959). "Changes in blood of dogs and rabbit by high fat intakes." *Am. J. Physiol.* 196, p. 473.

Swank, R. L. (1951). "Changes in blood produced by a fat meal and by intravenous heparin." *Am. J. Physiol.* 164, p. 798.

Swank, R. L. (1954). "Effect of high fat feedings on viscosity of the blood." *Science* 120, p. 427.

Swank, R. L. (1956). "Effect of fat on blood viscosity in dogs." *Circ. Res.* 4, p. 579.

Swank, R. L. (1962). "The influence of ecologic factors on blood, viscosity and sedimentation and on serum cholesterol." *Am. J. Clin. Nutr.* 10, p. 418.

Teitel, P. (1971). "A hemorheological view on molecular interaction between red blood cell constituents in the pathogenesis of constitutional hemolytic anemias." *Haematologia* 5, (1–2), p. 37.

Thomas, H. W. (1962). "The wall effect in capillary instruments: An improved analysis suitable for application to blood and other particulate suspensions." *Biorheology* 1, p. 41.

Thomas, H. W., R. J. French, A. C. Groom, and S. Rowlands (1965). "The flow of red cell suspensions through narrow tubes: The (extracorporeal) determination of the difference in mean velocities of red cells and their suspending phase." In *Symposium on Biorheology*, A. L. Copley (Ed.), (1965), p. 381.

Thomas, H. W. and D. E. Janes (1966). "The trapped supernatant in the packed red cell column on centrifugation of bovine red cell suspensions and its relation to the deformability of the red cell." In *Hemorheology*, A. L. Copley (Ed.), (1968), p. 569.

Thorsen, G. and H. Hint (1950). "Aggregation, sedimentation and intravascular sludging of erythrocytes." *Acta Chim. Scand. Suppl.* 154, p. 1.

Thurston, G. B. (1972). "Viscoelasticity of human blood." *Biophysical J.* 12, p. 1205.

Thurston, G. (1972). "Frequency and shear rate dependency of viscoelasticity of human blood." First International Congress of Biorheology, Lyon, France, September 1972.

Tibblin, G., S. E. Bergertz, J. Bjure, and L. Wilhelmson (1966). "Hematocrit, plasma, protein, plasma volume and viscosity in early hypertensive disease." *Am. Heart J.* 72, p. 165.

Tichner, E. G. and A. H. Sacks (1971). "Simulation studies of blood flow through stenosis in microcirculation." *Microvasc. Res.* 3, p. 337.

Tichner, E. G. and A. H. Sacks (1967). "A theory for the static elastic behavior of blood vessels." *Biorheology* 4, p. 151.

Tillich, G., L. Mendoza, H. Wayland, and R. J. Bing (1971). "Studies of the coronary microcirculation of the cat." *Am. J. Cardiol.* 27, p. 93.

Tollert, H. (1954). "Die Wirkung der Magnus-Kraft auf Sedimenterende teilchen Schuttinger sowie auf laminar Stromende und Gasgemische." *Naturwiss.* 41, p. 277.

Trap-Jensen, J. and N. A. Lassen (1970). Capillary permeability for smaller hydrophilic tracers in exercising skeletal muscle in normal man and in patients with long term diabetes melitus. In *Capillary Permeability*, C. Crone and N. A. Lassen (Eds.). Munksgaard, Copenhagen, p. 135.

Trevan, J. W. (1918). "The viscosity of blood." *Biochem. J.* 12, p. 60.

Usami, S. and S. Chien (1972). "Shear deformation of red cell ghosts." First International Conference in Biorheology Lyon, France, September 1972.

Usami, S., S. Chien, and M. Gregersen (1971). "Hemoglobin solution as a plasma expander: Effects on blood viscosity." *Proc. Soc. Exp. Biol. Med.* 136, p. 1232.

Usami, S., S. Chien, and M. Gregersen (1971). "Viscometric behavior of young and aged erythrocytes." In *Theoretical and Clinical Hemorheology*. H. Hartert and A. L. Copley (Eds.), (1971), p. 266.

Uzsoy, N. K. (1964). "Cardiovascular findings in patients with sickle-cell anemia." *Am. J. Cardiol.* 13, p. 320.

Vand, V. (1948). "Viscosity of solutions and suspensions." *J. Phys. Colloid Chem.* 62, p. 277.

VanWazer, J. R., J. W. Lyons, K. Y. Kim, and R. T. Colwell (1963). *Viscosity and Flow Measurement*. Interscience, New York, p. 201.

Vargas, F. and J. A. Johnson (1964). "An estimate of reflection coefficients for rabbit heart capillaries." *J. Gen. Physiol.* 47, p. 667.

Vejlens, G. (1964). "The velocity distribution in suspension flowing through narrow tubes." *2nd Europ. Conf. Microcirc. – Bibl. Anat.* 4, p. 46.

Vejlens, G. (1938). "The distribution of leucocytes in the vascular system." *Diss. Acta Pathol. Microbiol. Scand.* Suppl. 23, p. 159.

Vidabaek, A. (1950). "Polycythemia vera: Course and prognosis." *Acta Med. Scand.* 138, p. 179.

Virgilio, R. W., D. M. Lang, E. D. Mundth, and J. E. McLenathan (1964). "The effect of temperature and hematocrit on the viscosity of blood." *Surgery* 55, p. 825.

Volger, E., H. Klose, and H. Schmid-Schönbein (1972). "The effect of reduced salinity on red cell aggregation: A model of aggregate formation." First International Conference of Biorheology, Lyon, France, September 1972.

Vuopio, P. and A. Eisalo (1964). "Hematocrit values in men with myocardial infarction." *Ann. Med. Int. Fenn.* 53, p. 39.

Walker, A. R. P. (1963). "Hematocrit, hemoglobin level, and coronary heart disease in the South African Bantu." *Am. Heart J.* 66, p. 283.

Wallentin, I. (1966). "Importance of tissue pressure for the fluid equilibrium between the vascular and interstitial compartments in the small intestine." *Acta Physiol. Scand.* 68, p. 304.

Wasserman, L. R. and H. S. Gilbert (1966). "Complications of polycythemia vera." *Sem. Hematol.* 3, p. 199.

Watanabe, T., S. Oaka, and M. Yamamoto (1963). "A phenomenological theory of the sigma effect." *Biorheology* 1, p. 193.

Watson, W. C. (1957). "Lipemia, heparin and blood viscosity." *Lancet* 273, p. 366.

Wayland, H. (1967). "Rheology and the microcirculation." *Gastroenterology* 52, p. 342.

Weale, F. E. (1967). *An Introduction to Surgical Hemodynamics.* Year Book Medical Publishers, Chicago, p. 59.

Weaver, J. P. A., A. Evans, and D. N. Walder (1969). "The effect of increased fibrinogen content on the viscosity of blood." *Clin. Sci.* 36, p. 1.

Weed, R. L., P. L. LaCelle, and E. W. Merrill (1969). "Metabolic dependence of red cell deformability." *J. Clin. Invest.* 48, p. 795.

Weed, R. (1970). "The importance of erythrocyte deformability." *Am. J. Med.* 49, p. 147.

Weibel, E. R. and D. M. Gomez (1962). "The architecture of the human lung." *Science* 137, p. 3530.

Wells, R. E. (1965). "The effects of plasma proteins upon the rheology of blood in microcirculation." *Symposium on Biorheology*, Part 4, A. L. Copley (Ed.), (1965), p. 431.

Wells, R. E. (1966). "Hemorheologic effects of the dextrans on erythrocyte aggregation: Hemodilution versus disaggregation." In *Hemorheology*, A. L. Copley (Ed.), (1968), p. 415.

Wells, R. E., E. R. Schildkraut, and H. E. Edgerton (1966). "Blood flow in the microvasculature of the conjunctiva in man." *Science* 151, p. 995.

Wells, R. E. (1967). "Blood flow in the microcirculation of man and the flow properties of blood: A correlative study." *Bibl. Anat.* 9, p. 520.

Wells. R. E., Jr. (1964). "Rheology of blood in the microvasculature." *N. Eng. J. Med.* 270, p. 832.

Wells, R. E., Jr. and E. W. Merrill (1962). "Influence of flow properties of blood upon viscosity – Hematocrit relationships." *J. Clin. Invest.* 41, p. 1591.

Wells, R. E., Jr., T. H. Gawronski, P. J. Cox, and R. D. Perera (1964). "Influence of fibrinogen on flow properties of erythrocyte suspensions." *Am. J. Physiol.* 207, p. 1035.

Wells, R. E., Jr. and E. W. Merrill (1961). "The variability of blood viscosity." *Am. J. Med.* 31, p. 505.

West, G. B. (1968). "Local humoral factors influencing the microcirculation in shock." In *Micorcirculation as Related to Shock*, D. Shepro and G. P. Fulton (Eds.). Academic Press, New York, p. 149.

Whalen, W. J., J. Riley, and P. Nair (1967). "Microelectrode for measuring intracellular pO_2." *J. Appl. Physiol.* 23, p. 798.

Whitaker, S. R. F. and F. R. Winton (1933). "The apparent viscosity of blood flowing in the isolated hind limb of the dog and its variation with corpuscular concentration." *J. Physiol.* 78, p. 339.

Whitmore, R. L. (1963). "Hemorheology and hemodynamics." *Biorheology* 1, p. 201.

Whitmore, R. L. (1967). "A theory of blood flow in small vessels." *J. Appl. Physiol.* 22 (4), p. 767.

Whitmore, R. L. (1968). *Rheology of the Circulation.* Pergamon Press, Oxford, p. 93.

Wiedeman, M. P. (1962). "Lengths and diameters of peripheral arterial vessels in the living animal." *Circ. Res.* 10, p. 686.

Wiedeman, M. P. (1963). "Dimensions of blood vessels from distributing artery to collecting vein." *Circ. Res.* 12, p. 375.

Wiederhielm, C. A. (Ed.) (1966). "Quantitative methods for investigating the microcirculation." In *Methods in Medical Research*, Vol. 2, R. F. Rushmer (Ed.), Year Book Medical Publishers, Chicago, p. 42.

Wiederhielm, C. A. (1963). "Continuous recording of arteriolar dimensions with a television microscope." *J. Appl. Physiol.* 18, p. 1041.

Wiederhielm, C. A., J. W. Woodbury, S. Kink, and R. F. Rushmer (1964). "Pulsatile pressures in the microcirculation of the frog's mesentary." *Am. J. Physiol.* 207, p. 173.

Wiederhielm, C. A. (1965). "Viscoelastic properties of relaxed and constricted arteriolar walls." *3rd Europ. Conf. Microcirc., Jerusalem, 1964 — Bibl. Anat.* 7, p. 346, Karger, Basel/New York.

Wiederhielm, C. A. (1968). "Capillary fluid exchange." In *Biological Interface Flows and Exchanges. Proceedings of a Symposium Sponsored by the New York Heart Association.* Little, Brown, Boston.

Wiener, B. and A. Silberberg (1968). "A model for transcapillary flow." Abstracted in *5th Europ. Conf. on Microcirc.,* Gothenburg, Sweden.

Wilkinson, W. L. (1960), *Non-Newtonian Flow.* Pergamon Press, New York, p. 28.

Williams, A. R. (1972). "Hydrodynamic disruption of human erythrocytes." First International Conference of Biorheology, Lyon France, September 1972.

Williams, A. V., A. C. Higginbotham, and M. H. Knisely (1957). "Increased blood cell agglutination following ingestion of fat, a factor contributing to cardiac ischemia, coronary insufficiency and anginal pain." *Angiology* 8, p. 29.

Williams, R. C., Jr. (1968). "Hyperviscosity syndromes." *Circulation* 38, p. 450.

Winslow, C. E. A. and L. P. Herrington (1949). *Temperature and Human Life.* Princeton University Press, Princeton, N.J. Cited from *Exercise Physiology*, H. B. Falls (Ed.). Academic Press, New York, 1968, p. 196.

Wintrobe, N. M. (1962). *Clinical Hematology*, Lea & Febiger, Philadelphia, p. 323.

Zander, R. and H. Schmid-Schönbein (1972). "Oxygen release of human erythrocytes during flow." Seventh Conference of Microcirculation, Aberdeen, Scotland. (Abstract).

Zimmerman, S. L. and H. Barnet (1944). "Sickle-cell anemia simulating coronary occulsion." *Ann. Int. Med.* 21, p. 1045.

Zoll, P. M., S. Wessler, and M. J. Schlesinger (1951). "Interarterial coronary anastamoses in the human heart with particular reference to anemia and relative cardiac anoxia." *Circulation* 4, p. 797.

Zoll. P. M. and L. R. Norman (1952). "The effects of vasomotor drugs and of anemia on coronary anastomoses." *Circulation* 6, p. 832.

Zweifach, B. W. (1961). *Functional Behavior of the Microcirculation.* Charles C. Thomas, Springfield, Ill.

Zweifach, B. W. and M. Intaglietta (1968). "Mechanism of fluid movement across single capillaries in the rabbit." *Microvasc. Res.* 1, p. 83.

Zweifach, B. W. and M. Intaglietta (1971). "Measurement of blood plasma colloid osmotic pressure. II. Comparative study of different species." *Microvasc. Res.* 3, p. 83.

Index